# ULTIMATE SURVIVORSHIP
## The Breast Cancer Manual

CHRISTINE ANDERSON

The information included in this book is for educational purposes only. It is neither intended nor implied to be a substitute for professional medical advice. You should *always* consult your healthcare provider to determine the appropriateness of any information for your own situation or if you have any questions regarding your medical condition or treatment plan. Further, you should not undertake any changes in your diet or exercise patterns without first consulting your doctor.

The information provided is solely intended to be used by you and your medical team in creating a treatment plan that is most suitable for your specific situation and as a springboard to ask questions of your doctor; it references the scientific work of researchers and nutritionists, which may be reviewed at www.ultimatesurvivorship.com/resources/references.

Finally, please note that, for simplicity's sake, I have chosen to use female pronouns throughout the book. I do understand that there are men with breast cancer and that we often have male doctors. I am using this convention solely to avoid the repeated use of "he or she."

www.ultimatesurvivorship.com
christine@ultimatesurvivorship.com

ISBN-10: 0615960561

ISBN-13: 978-0615960562

## DEDICATION

For my daughters, Katie Anne and Rachel Jane,
and for the best friend a girl could ever hope for, Irene.

I love you so.

# CONTENTS

PHASE TWO: THE LIFESTYLE

# ACKNOWLEDGMENTS

I would like to acknowledge the love and support of all of the wild and wise women in my life, including head cheerleaders Irene Gates, Beth Keltz, Arlene Ninke Barber, Jeannie Sanders, Susan Kuite-Smith, and Lisa Silver-Cassidy, and of my hubby Mike Anderson, and daughter Rachel Morrissett. Without each of you here with me, everything would be much, much more difficult and my path a thousand times less beautiful. And way less interesting.

I will never, as long as I live, forget the grace, generosity, and kindness of an army of breast cancer survivors who came to walk at my side in small and large ways, who shared their lives, their stories, their strength, and their wisdom, including my high school buddy Debby Ramey Burnett and new friends Mary Stellick and Chris Gonzales, and so many more. Your presence in my life is a gift, and I will spend the rest of my life paying your generosity of spirit forward.

Sincere thanks to manuscript readers who offered suggestions and went over my writing at various stages of production, including extra-special readers extraordinaire Bridget Allen, Heather Greig, and Marla Wedge, who did a brilliant job of polishing this whole thing up when the rest of us had eyes that were bleary with words, words, and more words; and to my brother, Andrew Greig, for assistance getting the artwork to the finish line.

I would most especially like to acknowledge the help of the dedicated and incomparable Erfert Fenton and Kimberly Allen, two generous and amazing women without whose skillful editing this book truly would not have come into being. I also extend my sincere thanks to the talented writer Mark Canter for sharing his gift with the world and what he knows about making books with me.

I give my undying gratitude to Dr. Leon Oostendorp in Grand Rapids, the breast cancer surgeon who personally called me with the good news that he got it all the first time. And to my oncology care team at Cancer Treatment Centers of America in Chicago, headed by the amazing Dr. Kaoutar Tlemcani: I thank you from the bottom of my heart. You are all the very embodiment of patient-centered medical care.

This is my village.

# PHASE ONE: THE NEWS

Gathering your wits about you,
building your teams,
getting your duckies all in a row,
and making really big decisions.

*"You must do the thing you think you cannot do."*

~ Eleanor Roosevelt

# 1. YOUR BODY IS NOT A BATTLEFIELD

Okay, let me be perfectly honest: I very selfishly wrote this book just for me. This is the how-to manual I searched in vain for in the days and weeks after I was diagnosed with early stage breast cancer, the book that would tell me exactly how to do this thing I was completely unprepared to do, beginning day one and guiding me through the rest of my life.

To be more clear: I researched this book for me because I could find absolutely nothing like it anywhere. A year and a half later I put it all in writing for someone I love dearly. And now, I share the wealth of information I've gathered with all of you, my sisters who have joined me on the same challenging path.

On January 11, 2011, at 1PM, I got a call from my doctor that gave me an all-access, all-hours pass into the club that no one wants to be in. Chances are, if you're reading this, you've heard the same words I did that day: "I am sorry to have to give you this news. Your biopsy was positive. You have breast cancer." I have breast cancer. I have breast cancer? What?! Are you freaking serious?!?! My brain began to buzz with the immense word cancer cancercancercancercancercancercancercancercancercancercancercanc ercancercancercancercancercancercancercancercancercancercancerca ncercancercancercancercancercancercancercancercancercancercancer cancercancercancercancercancercancercancercancercancercancercanc ercancercancercancercancercancercancercancercancercancercancer.

And in that tiny slice of time, in that infinitesimal moment in the 54-year-long science experiment known as my life, for the first time ever, I experienced paralyzing, gut-wrenching, sucker-punch, drop-me-to-my knees fear, literally unable to draw oxygen into my lungs. It was several minutes before I could feel anything but utter panic . . . and when that finally subsided, I began to weep. Out loud and in living color. Mike had just left to run errands, and once I thought I had composed myself enough to speak, I called him . . . but when I heard his voice, my throat closed again and I could get nothing more than a few choked sobs out.

And so it began.

Once the initial shock wore off, I started making The Calls. I know you know what I'm talking about—calls to everyone that matters in our known universe to give notice that life has just changed. Forever. If you knew me, you'd know that I do not like to talk on the telephone, especially since all I have is a cell phone, and it gets hot after a few minutes, and I hate that. The second-of-all was that I was already, with less than a week of being diagnosed with breast cancer under my belt, emotionally spent from saying the same things over and over.

And so, I started processing in the only way I know how. For me, that means researching and reading and asking questions, and always, always, writing: I started a little blog for those closest to me, My Body is Not a Battlefield, and shared not only appointments, but pictures, thoughts, and experiences, as I made my way through treatment.

The tumor was at 11:00, deep, near my chest wall. If you look at my right breast as a clock. Which I never did before. So there was a serious paradigm shift right there. The first of many.

I remember being spectacularly overwhelmed with all of the thoughts, crazy and sane, banging around in my brain, and trying to perform some kind of a sort-out, and jeez Louise, there is a lot of freaking information that needs to be relayed to a lot of people, and a lot of stuff to figure out, and where do I start? Should I get a good planner set up so I can organize all of my doctor appointments and papers? Will I lose my job from being off work too much and end up living in a tepee in the woods? Will I be able to work and still do my treatments? Am I saying too much to people that don't know me very well? Will I lose my hair, and if I do, can I please tell everyone that I love that I do not want them to think they all hafta shave their heads so I'm not so goofy-looking all by myself? What does this mean? What does that stand for? What does that mean? Will my insurance cover this? Am I going to die? Am I going to die? Am I going to fucking die? Yeah, that's the big one, the big scary furry creature that sat in a chair across the room from me in the first days and weeks of knowing I had cancer, waiting for me to look over there and acknowledge its big creepy presence, or at least wanting to make me cry, again, again, all the time sitting there staring at me with its big stinky armpits filling the room with the odor of fear since the moment I got that call.

In those first weeks of waiting and wondering, I wasn't able to avoid the scenarios that I played and replayed in my mind over what might happen. I experienced the full intensity of human emotion, and not just the horrible, gut-twisting ones. So many people quietly moved in to stand at my side, and I experienced the enormous blessing of knowing just how much I am loved, and by whom, while I was still around to appreciate it.

What the heck, when I wrote "people" just there, I should have written "women." Because although I have a wonderfully supportive and loving husband, men-friends to whom my continued existence matters at least a little bit, and a father who loves me a bunch, it was the women that came to my emotional rescue, doing one of the many things we do exceptionally well: Giving love, and always, unconditional support.

One woman-friend told me, "Wrap yourself in the armor of love and take courage," and with that mantra inscribed on my heart, I was able to face many a difficult day. Another reminded me that a burden shared is a burden divided, and yet another told me she would make me a turban if I lost my hair.

I wondered: Did they have someone reach out to them the way they did to me? I swore that I would do the same someday, and that I would never forget their grace and kindness.

Many told me that I was strong. Most days, that's true, but I have to tell you that there are times, even now, fully in remission, when I am not strong at all: Sometimes I am a blubbering mess. And I am also fully aware that this disease has taken many strong women. But I know what was meant, what was intended, when they said that, and I know why they did, and so I reframed the message: Christine, remember to be strong.

> Women I didn't even know came rushing to whisper their secrets in my ear, women ahead of me on this same path, holding me gently at each elbow. I wondered: Did they have someone reach out to them the way they did to me? I swore that I would do the same someday, and that I would never forget their grace and kindness.

So many reminded me to laugh, to take deep breaths, to decide how I wanted to move forward. Another suggested I write my own Cancer Rules for Friends and Family. I never did that, but the idea made me smile. (And still seems like a great idea. Christine's Rule Number One: When you are talking to me, your friend who has recently been diagnosed with breast cancer, do not tell me stories about people who died of cancer. Argh! And I am telling you, that happens. A lot.)

The best laugh in those early days was a tee shirt one woman was wearing at a fundraising event, upon which she had written, "Of course they're fake. My real ones tried to kill me!" I find such beauty in her ability to create humor in something I know to be a painful and often terrifying place.

Mike and I kept busy with fun things, and we spent time holding hands and talking. I also continued running every day, because I could, and I ran in gratitude for that. I deepened my meditation practice. I consciously tried to remember to open my chest and to breathe, especially outdoors. And I intentionally remembered to take note of all of the beauty I am immersed in, the natural beauty that is the land shaped like a hand, my beloved Michigan, lakeshore and woods.

I asked my best friend in the whole wide world, Irene, to give me a haircut in preparation for maybe losing my hair completely one day soon. For those who don't know, we've been best friends since we met in the ninth grade, in the girls' bathroom at the new junior high. (And that, my dears, was 43 years ago.) She is a hysterically funny Cajun lady, a gifted artist, and she was pretty shook up about this whole cancer deal in general.

I was the last haircut of the day in a small beauty shop in our little Midwestern town, and when she was done we sat and drank a couple of mochas and talked and laughed and cried and hugged and talked some more and then cried some more. Right before I left we laughed so hard about something that the people in the shop next door must have thought we were nuts. So that was a good time to go home.

All in all, I don't believe I'd like to live in a world that doesn't have Irene in it. I cannot even conjure what that might look like, which makes the fact that she, too, was recently diagnosed with breast cancer practically impossible to process. Unlike me, she is not one to tell the world all of her business, and so I will leave it at that.

And I made one huge decision: My body is not a battlefield. This battlefield idea is a metaphor with great power for a great many people, and I respect that, but for me, as a lover and a peacemaker, I cannot wrap myself around the idea that I am waging war against myself, in my very own body.

I hope against all hope that once you have read this book from beginning to end, you will join me in making this paradigm shift, that you will join me in seeing the process of recovery and ultimate survivorship not as an act of war, but as an act of ultimate self-love.

This thing that grew inside me came from within me . . . it was not an outside invader, it was my very own cells and it was giving me clues that I needed to follow to their source. And so I did. I asked questions of my conventional medical team, well-respected oncologists and nurses to a fault, about diet and exercise and the mind-body connections to help me deal with my treatment and diagnosis.

I was answered with little more than quizzical expressions. (Until I found the clinic that is now my home. No more quizzical expressions!) These were specialists with years of training and experience, including oncology nurses and dietitians, people whose job it is to know the biology of cancer, and they, for the most part, thought I was just a little too serious in this line of questioning.

Please do not misunderstand any of what I just wrote as lack of respect for the men and women who have dedicated their lives to doctoring cancer patients. I love conventional medicine. It is the foundation of my treatment plan, designed by me and my medical team.

I trust that the day is coming in which conventional medicine will automatically include the aspects that I have also woven into my treatment plan without a patient being required to demand it as I have. Contemporary scientific inquiry is showing us the way: There is more to the eradication of breast cancer than just aiming big guns at it. (But I like big guns too.)

Onward and upward. Tears cried, fear faced squarely, and with all of these thoughts swirling in my mind, I continued to learn as much as I could about this thing that was happening in my body. I decided to figure out how to live a statistically longer life, how to give myself every shot in the world of being an old lady, and, my friends, not just any old lady, but a truly joyful old broad who can't wait for whatever is gonna happen next because she knows it's gonna be absolutely amazing.

> My body is not a battlefield. This battlefield idea is a fine metaphor with great power for a great many people, and I respect that, but for me, as a lover and a peacemaker, I cannot wrap myself around the idea that I am waging war against myself, in my very own body.

Bit by bit I learned new things about breast cancer, ways to make sure that I never have to do this again, ways to cope with the emotional upheaval that had just plopped itself down right-smack in the middle of my life.

I committed myself to research, making sure to pay attention to information that was backed up by good science. I read, and I read, and I read some more. I took notes. I asked questions. I listened to women who spoke from their experience.

And I began to change my life in amazing ways I never could have even dreamed just months before.

Make no mistake: I acknowledge moments of fear that creep up from behind when I least expect it. I give this fear space from time to time, and in my opinion, there has been nothing quite as liberating as contemplating the distinct possibility of my own death—allowing me to magnify the incredible beauty of being here just one more day.

And so, fear is given space, allowed to co-exist with the dead-calm confident knowledge that everything is exactly as it needs to be.

This book is not simply about sharing how I learned to take charge of my breast cancer treatment, although that's absolutely and positively the first thing that I want you to know, and the belief from which all others spring. It's not simply about increasing your chances of joining the burgeoning ranks of women enjoying long-term survival after a breast cancer diagnosis, although that's certainly a huge part of what we are aiming for, when it all boils down to the nitty-gritty of the thing. This is about taking charge of the quality of the rest of your life, about living life joyfully, intentionally, and yes, out loud, no matter what.

This is my opportunity—literally a step-by-step plan—to give as many women as possible the head start I wasn't given as I struck out on the single most challenging and confusing journey of my life, as a breast cancer survivor, a journey that began the moment I heard the terrifying news.

There are so many things we have no control over as we walk this path, but there are far more that we do, and I would like to share with you the things that I have learned. The words I am putting on these pages are part of what I can do to pay it forward, to honor the grace and kindness I have been shown, and continue to be shown to this very day.

This is your journey, and I fervently hope that it begins in earnest, and with joyful intention, today. It's time to feed your mind, embrace and fuel your body, and nurture your spirit.

Peace to you, my dear sisters. I'm so glad you're here. Let's get started!

# 2. TAKE CHARGE

Breast cancer is a gigantic, all-encompassing, life-changing diagnosis, and more than a little intimidating. There's a metric ton of information out there and much of it is simply not worth our time. Everyone (and their mother) has thoughts on What You Should Do, and the choices that abound are confusing at best.

Add to that the fact that no two breast cancers are exactly alike: Each has its own genetic fingerprint and may respond differently to proposed therapies. One more gargantuan thing to throw into the mix is most certainly the emotional component: Having cancer is scary!

The medical community is beginning to understand how complicated and frightening a breast cancer diagnosis can be, and there are now "nurse navigators" being utilized in many practices who will help you keep track of things and who will make themselves available to answer questions.

That's awesome, but in spite of that, it is critically important for you to remember this: There is no one in this whole wide world who will be a better advocate, or a better friend to you, than *you*.

*Become an active participant*

My step two, take charge, means empowering yourself to demand better care by becoming an active participant in the process of developing your treatment plan rather than a passive bystander who simply shuffles from one treatment to the next without any real understanding of the magnitude of what is happening in (and to) your body.

This is a big deal here! There are lifelong ramifications to the therapies you will be considering shortly. It's a spectacular time to really pay attention to what's going on around you.

The practice of oncology is often as much an art as it is a science. It is an exciting and fast-moving discipline with breakthroughs taking place at lightning pace. There will be times during your treatment when you will have to decide what to do next and there will be no roadmap other than what you have laid on your heart and what you have decided to do.

When my tumor was sent out for analysis, it came back labeled an intermediate risk for recurrence. I had to make a decision based on what was important to me and how I wanted to live my life. I made the decision to focus on taking excellent care of myself, increasing the odds that the tumor would not recur after surgery with an improved lifestyle as I've described in these pages, and without the assistance of chemotherapy.

By the way, the story I just told isn't a lesson that says, "Don't choose chemo." Instead, it's a way to illustrate that what you want is what the doctors need to do. The lesson in this story says, "This belongs to you and no one else." I had made the decision long before the test came back that I would go through chemo if I thought it was necessary, and I decided that it wasn't. Do not let anyone decide anything for you. If there is anything in this entire epic that I mean with every fiber of my being it is: This is your journey. No one else's. You are the decider.

That said, this *is not* to say you should do this without a doctor, making up your treatment based on articles you have read on the internet. We must go through treatment with a breast cancer oncologist on the medical team! You will find that I advocate in these pages for finding a doctor who is up to running speed with the current evidence on nutrition, exercise, and lifestyle choices, but an oncologist it must be.

And this is not simply about demanding better care. It's also about being able to hold up your end of the bargain in a doctor-patient relationship in a meaningful way. Trust me, a good oncologist (or a good nurse, or a good nutritionist, or . . . well, you catch my drift) will be thrilled to know that you understand what she is talking about and that you really do have insight into the options that are on the table, or that you even might have an option of your own that you'd like to discuss. If she is not thrilled, well, I say it's time to look for a new doctor.

When we go into that little examination room with one of the people on our oncology team, we only get a few minutes to receive and understand information *from* as well as to effectively and confidently relay information *to* the professional we are meeting with. A prepared patient who is paying attention and understands the terminology can ask good questions, in order to receive even better information, and receive even better care.

While it doesn't happen often, a patient who has placed herself in charge and is thus paying attention will have a much greater ability to notice when mistakes are being made. Doctors may be well trained, but they do make mistakes from time to time, and I can assure you from personal experience that medical bureaucratic systems are not always in good working order. One person in the oncology practice who is not doing her job can result in a mistake that could affect you in tremendous ways for a very long time.

For example, my initial diagnosis was held up for weeks by a lost film that the radiologist needed in order to complete the report. Because of a high-risk history, I was supposed to get digital mammograms and ultrasounds every six months. The hospital called the day before a scheduled mammogram to tell me that they couldn't go ahead with the appointment because the clinic had not returned the films from six months before. I contacted the clinic and was assured that the hospital had made an error, so I called the hospital, and they looked around again. Still no films.

The day of the mammo appointment came. And went, without me. Along came another regularly scheduled appointment at the clinic (no mammogram or ultrasound in hand, obviously). I asked once again if they could look for my films. The physician's assistant personally went and looked for them. Nowhere on the premises. She guaranteed it.

Finally, I called the hospital in a state of desperation and told them I *had* *to* have a mammogram and ultrasound whether they could find the films or not. If I had to start from scratch, so be it. Fast forward to mammogram results: Abnormal film and ultrasound showing a possibly cancerous lesion. People, the radiologist was unable to complete the report without the comparison films.

> The practice of oncology is often as much an art as it is a science.

And I was waiting to hear if I had cancer! Phone calls, phone calls, phone calls. A biopsy ensued with the full report still incomplete pending missing film. Finally, one of the radiology technicians in my itty-bitty local hospital made a last-ditch call to the clinic and spoke with someone (a clerk of some sort) who, within a few minutes, had located my films in a pile labeled "To Be Destroyed."

I am not joking! This was after two months of me (and the hospital) asking about them on a number of occasions . . . and being told repeatedly that they did not have them. No one had really looked. They had all simply assumed the films weren't there because they weren't *supposed* to be there. They had all just looked at a notation jotted in the file that said, "film returned to originating hospital," and considered it a done deal. I was by that time almost three months late on the diagnosis. I am glad I paid attention. I'm glad I was persistent. I am glad I had taken charge.

It is important to remember, then, that our doctors and nurses can only do so much for us. Doctors play a critical role in our medical care, but we absolutely must take our own health into our own hands and take responsibility for the way we take care of ourselves.

We have the power—no, the obligation!—to make better choices, realizing that the quality of our life isn't just about the medical community and what *they* can do for *us*. *We must rely upon ourselves* and trust that we know what is best for us, using the best medical information we can wrap our brains around.

Knowledge is power.

This would be a great place to acknowledge that not all women are comfortable taking charge in the way I have described. I'm not here to change your core personality or the way you do business if it causes you distress.

Some women have a more shy and unassertive nature and wouldn't be comfortable in that kind of a queen-of-the-universe role. That's perfectly okay, but in that instance, please make sure that there is someone on your support team who will be able to advocate for you in the way I have described.

## THE BOTTOM LINE

It is time to take charge, my sister, to understand what is happening in your body, to speak with confidence and authority about what needs to be done about it, to play an active role in your treatment, to rejoice in this amazing machine you stroll around in each and every day, and to live well, no matter the time that you are given, for, as we all know, there are no promises.

There are no promises.

# 3. SLOW DOWN: BREAST CANCER IS NOT (USUALLY) AN EMERGENCY

Now that you have set yourself up as the boss of this whole life-changing yet life-affirming, let's-get-rid-of-my-breast-cancer-please situation, it's time to slow down just a little. It is time to gather your wits about you as much as is possible, given the general impossibility of being calm after such a diagnosis is dished out.

There is (probably) going to be a fair amount of time that elapses between diagnosis and treatment, so use it to your advantage in a number of ways. Allow yourself the freedom to feel all of the emotions that rise to the surface without trying to tamp them down or smother them out. Cry, if that is what you need to do, and do it whenever you need to.

Don't judge anything you are thinking and for heaven's sake don't let anyone else judge your reactions or emotions either, no matter how well-meaning they believe they are. No one who hasn't had to deal with their very own personal cancer diagnosis could possibly have the slightest idea what it feels like to be standing in our shoes, brains on fire with possibilities and questions, and yes, sometimes even fear.

When I was first diagnosed (especially before I had any real information about the behavioral characteristics of my tumor) I wanted to talk about things I was afraid of, and Mike simply would not allow such talk. It wasn't until I had this exact conversation with my best friend that I realized any conversation my hubby and I engaged in that brought forth the simultaneous thoughts "Christine" and "death" was not a conversation he was willing to have. (And now I get it. Duh.)

When I tried to talk about my fears, he said I was being negative and alluded to the distinct possibility that I was inviting disaster into the situation when I voiced them. Silently, he was saying, "It's too scary to talk like this."

And like many husbands, he also wanted to fix it and tell me that everything was going to be just fine, and any other thoughts were simply not going to be entertained.

Thereafter, when I was feeling scared and needed to give voice to those quite natural thoughts, I either wrote, or called on any number of friends who I knew could safely handle the concept of me being scared of dying for a minute. I sometimes needed to say the frightening what-ifs out loud before I could let them go.

So. Slow it down and work your way through some of the tougher emotions with someone who can help you get through it. "Slow it down?! Slow it down, you say?! Are you kidding me?! I want this thing outta me! Now!" I hear that, and I get it, but I suppose now's as good a time as any to tell you what I learned right out of the gate, from one of my first nurses.

In a moment in which I was engulfed in absolute panic about how slow things seemed to be moving, she calmly commented to me, "Sweetheart, don't take this wrong, but cancer isn't usually a medical emergency." Despite our personal and quite profound opinion to the contrary, we typically have plenty of time to figure things out.

### How old is your tumor?

I believe this might also be the perfect place to talk about how long you have probably had breast cancer, quietly growing: Hidden, happy, warm and well-nourished in the sweet chemical soup that is so perfectly and adorably you.

The normal, healthy cells that make up everything in and out of our bodies grow and divide, become injured or old, and die a natural cell death, becoming absorbed by our bodies. This is the cycle of biological life for all living things. Cancer cells, however, operate in an entirely different way when it comes to natural cell death: They don't die. They just keep growing and dividing, growing and dividing, until eventually they become a big enough mass to refer to as a tumor.

"How long has this tumor been growing, then?" you may ask. Good question, and one of many I asked, myself, during Phase One of The Great Breast Cancer Eradication Project. And so, here are a few facts on that particular topic.

Based on data from over 3,000 patients in five different studies, researchers found the median recurrence rate of breast cancer that was not medically treated after the primary tumor was removed to be 2.7 years. By median, they are referring to that one patient in the exact middle of the pack: Half of the numbers were higher, and half were lower. Using numbers generated this way helped them to estimate that most breast cancers are five to six years old by the time they are large enough to be detected.

Dr. Michael Retsky, a leading authority on tumor growth, has also done similar calculations on breast tumor growth that support this estimate. Dr. Retsky states that a single breast cancer cell, growing by simple cell division, has divided approximately 30 times before it is easily detectable at one centimeter, half the width of a penny, which is roughly the size of my tumor when it was first detected by digital mammography.

I never was able to feel my tumor, even after I knew it was there, because it lay deep in my breast, near the chest wall, and to further complicate things, I have dense breasts and numerous cysts. My oncologist doubts that I would have noticed it on my own until it was much larger.

Dr. Retsky concluded that each cell division takes between 25 and 1,000 days, with a "typical" rate that ages most breast cancer tumors at two to five years by the time they are noticed.

## THE BOTTOM LINE

Breast cancer treatment isn't necessarily determined simply by the age or size of the tumor, making it, honestly, not always particularly relevant to treatment decisions. So why go through all of these explanations, then? To help you understand a little more clearly why my nurse told me that breast cancer is not an emergency, to allow you to realize that you must slow down and gather yourself together, and to gain a whole new perspective on the time element of breast cancer treatment.

While treatment decisions aren't something that should take weeks and weeks, it is, generally speaking, imperative that you not rush any decisions about your treatment. Or panic about how ridiculously long everything seems to be taking. Take a deep breath.

# 4. LEARN TO BREATHE

Our lives, yours and mine, are changed in myriad ways, and forever. Our days are now ordered by appointments to be kept, records to maintain, insurance to be overseen . . . and all of this on top of everything else that we currently juggle in our busy lives. If we allow it, stress and tension can take control. It doesn't need to be that way.

A number of mind-body techniques will be introduced in a few chapters, but for right now, let's talk about one of the simplest ways to change the direction of your day, from chaos and stress to calm intention: Breathing. It's ridiculously easy, it's something we all do approximately 20,000 times a day, without even noticing, and it is a gift that we can harness as a powerful mood-changer when the going gets tough.

Let's start here: What happens when we are feeling stressed? (Stressed, like maybe when we have been recently diagnosed with cancer, for example?) Nestled deep in our brains is a small neurostructure, the amygdala, a powerful buddy that has the ability to immediately interrupt thought and physical processes by releasing hormones into the bloodstream: Adrenaline, noradrenaline, epinephrine, and norepinephrine.

These in turn rush around with the task of jumpstarting a variety of physiological reactions. Your heart rate speeds up, you breathe harder and faster, your blood and metabolic rates rise, blood flows to your muscles. Your pupils dilate so you can focus on the danger at hand. Lung bronchi dilate to assist with blood oxygenation and to convert energy stored in the liver into fuel for strength and endurance. Time to giddy-up GO!

Hundreds of centuries ago, when these systems and responses were evolving, they served us well and kept us alive in an environment where hypervigilance was a necessity. Known as the "fight-or-flight" response, it's what allowed us to hit the road at a moment's notice, or stay and fight if running away wasn't an option. I imagine it oftentimes really was a matter of running fast, throwing a rock, or being eaten.

This tiny almond-shaped structure that jumpstarts all of these systems is a super-sensitive, hair-trigger instrument, tied to both hemispheres of the brain and paying close attention to even the tiniest details of our thoughts and bodily responses to the environment around us. The amygdala is the security system of the human anatomy.

The good news is that we do not have to be held at the mercy of this hypervigilant little brain-almond. The nature of the thoughts we choose, as sages throughout time have known, have a profound effect on how our physical body responds when confronted by the unavoidable stressors associated with life, including a cancer diagnosis and the treatment that follows. We do not have to be swept away by our emotions, which, left unchecked, can take a terrible toll on us both emotionally and physically.

There is a deep, mysterious, and intimate relationship between our mind and body that we have only just begun to explore scientifically. The wisest among us have always taught that a person's breath will automatically respond to even the minutest cues from the brain. It will adjust in depth and speed according to our thoughts and feelings. Our bodies hear and respond to everything we are thinking: Stressed breathing tends to be shallower, faster, and can actually prolong feelings of anxiety.

We have the ability to create a sense of well-being in the midst of all of this chaos. We can stop the fight-or-flight response in its tracks and instead trigger the initiation of an entirely different chemical response that is led by endorphin production, all by the power of our minds, and with the assistance of intentional breathing. This type of slow breathing will actually stimulate the parasympathetic system, the system that works to calm us down.

Deepak Chopra, in his book, *Ageless Body, Timeless Mind*, stated, "Wherever a thought goes, a chemical goes with it." And so, we intentionally change our breathing pattern, we change the thought ever so slightly, and chemicals that stimulate a positive reaction in our bodies will be released, changing the moment in profound ways. We all have this power. We will explore several simple and effective mind-body techniques later on, but for now, let's simply focus on the breath.

There are as many variations on relaxation breathing techniques as there are people who practice them, but there are a few classic techniques that you can begin to utilize right away. There are some that you will find calming, some that you will find relaxing, and some energizing. I encourage you to try these basic techniques as soon as possible to find at least one that works well for you.

*Belly breathing*

Taking 10 deep belly breaths is perhaps one of the simplest, fastest ways to shift your mind and body into a calm(er) state of mind. Here's how:

- Sit comfortably with your spine straight.

- Exhale the air in your lungs completely.

- Inhale very, very slowly, allowing the breath to enter without extra force or effort, through your nose. While you are doing this, allow your abdomen to push out and rise. Try to move your chest as little as possible. Some people, if they are in a place where this is feasible, will lie down flat on their backs and place a light object on their abdomen so that there is a visual reminder that it is the tummy that rises up and down in this exercise, rather than the chest.

- After your abdomen has risen, allow your chest to rise and expand, allowing the middle part of your lungs to fill with air as well.

- Allow your abdomen to pull in ever so slightly, and allow your shoulders and collarbones to rise, which will fill the upper part of the lungs.

- Gently hold your breath for just a second or two. The key here is gently! Although you are not trying to force yourself to hold your breath in an uncomfortable way, gently stop in this place with lungs full of air and for the briefest of moments enjoy the feeling.

- Slowly begin to exhale through your nose. Breathe abdominally, pushing the air out of your lungs by contracting and tightening, pulling your abdominal muscles in as you release.

## *The 4-7-8 relaxing breath*

Dr. Andrew Weil highly recommends this breathing technique that stimulates a relaxation response. Weil refers to the 4-7-8 breathing technique as a "natural tranquilizer," suggesting that it will be a powerful tool to be used whenever you are beginning to feel upset or stressed. It is also a great way to fall asleep. Although you can do this exercise in any position, try to sit with your back straight while performing it, so as to have your chest open to receive its benefits.

- Begin by placing the tip of your tongue against the ridge of tissue just behind your upper front teeth, where it will stay while you are doing this exercise.

- Exhale gently, slowly, and completely, through your mouth. You will make an audible (though not loud) sound as you do this.

- Close your mouth. Inhale gently, slowly, and quietly, through your nose, to a count of *four*.

- Hold your breath for a count of *seven*.

- Exhale completely, through your mouth, again making an audible sound, this time for a count of *eight*.

- That process was one breath.

- Repeat the 4-7-8 cycle three more times, for a total of four repetitions.

You may have difficulty holding your breath for seven seconds, especially when you are just beginning to practice. You may (like me) find the act of holding your breath unpleasant. No worries. The number of seconds spent in each of the three phases is not as important as maintaining the relative ratio. In other words, your exhalation is twice as long as your inhalation, with the breath-holding portion just slightly under the length of exhalation.

Perform this exercise at least two times a day, and I guarantee that you will get deeper breaths over time. There's nothing that says you can't do it more often, but Weil suggests that you do not do more than four breaths at one time for the first month.

*Breath counting*

Another simple breathing technique, and good practice for meditation, is the simple act of breath counting. Wherever you are, whatever you are doing, begin by sitting comfortably and with a straight spine.

Close your eyes if this is at all possible. There are no special techniques in this exercise, just breathe in a calm and relaxed manner. Begin by taking a couple of deep, slow breaths. Now comes the hard part. Begin to count your breaths on the exhalation (in your mind, not out loud), but only up to five.

This deceptively simple technique will help you to remain calm and in the present. You will know that your attention has wandered when you suddenly realize that you have counted higher than five. Simply regain control of the counting, and begin again. Try to do this exercise for about ten minutes.

*Alternate nostril breathing (moon and sun breathing)*

I first learned about and practiced alternate nostril breathing in yoga class. I learned that in the natural, unaffected state of breathing during the course of a day, we don't always breathe through both nostrils: We tend to breathe out of one or the other. (I didn't know that, did you?)

Practitioners suggest that the left nostril corresponds to the parasympathetic system, the feminine, creative and lunar, while the right nostril corresponds to the sympathetic system, the male, hard-driving and solar.

The exercise that follows helps to balance the solar and the lunar, the feminine and the masculine, the yin and the yang. Yeah, that's all a bit esoteric, but I do know that (if nothing else) when I am feeling particularly stressed and distressed, this is the breathing technique I almost always engage.

Even if I am sitting somewhere where I can't do the hand-on-the-nose thing without people looking at me like I'm a bit nutty, I pretend in my mind's eye that I am, and visualize the air going where it needs to go for this exercise, and watch the sun and moon rise and set at my command. It's pretty awesome.

And you know what? There have been plenty of times when I have practiced this technique in the middle of a crowded waiting room, too. It was only necessary for me to take a few extra moments to find a quiet place inside me before beginning.

*The technique*

- Use your right thumb to close off the right nostril, and gently exhale.

- Slowly inhale through the left nostril.

- Pause ever so briefly.

- With right ring finger, close the left nostril.

- Exhale through your right nostril.

- Inhale through right nostril.

- Pause ever so briefly.

- Use thumb to close off right nostril.

- Breathe out through left nostril.

A modification of this technique involves visualizing the sun and moon rising and setting (moon rising on the left side, the sun on the right), and one other involves plugging your right nostril and taking 30 slow breaths just on the left side. Very calming.

The first time you try alternate nostril breathing, practice it for just one or two sequences and only gradually increase to more. When you are done, sit quietly for a minute or two. Honestly, it's not as tricky as it sounds, so give it a try. I find this method particularly calming and soothing. The image that always comes to mind when I am practicing this technique is the infinity symbol, which I believe to be a lovely thing for a cancer patient to be thinking about.

## THE BOTTOM LINE

No matter which intentional breathing technique you employ, I'm here to tell you that these are tremendous tools to have at your disposal, an almost sure-fire way to gather calm around you in even the most emotionally precarious situations. I realize it would be silly of me to suggest that breathing will solve all of your most pressing medical or emotional concerns, but I have found it to be a profoundly useful way to have a positive influence on my state of mind when I feel like things are about to fly apart.

# 5. BUILD A SUPPORT TEAM

Depending upon the complexity and intensity of the treatments you will be going through and what's on your plate in regard to family and job, it's possible that you're going to need some help making your way through this with your sanity intact. Sometimes I just wanted to be left alone to rest or write and other times I wanted to go kick up my heels and have a little bit of silly fun. I am fortunate to be blessed with an absolutely amazing network of girlfriends, near and far, who stepped in to give me exactly what was needed at just the right moment, time and time again.

There will be a number of people (friends, family, neighbors, social media buddies, and co-workers) who want to do something nice for you. Girlfriend, please allow them to do so. When someone asks, "Is there anything I can do for you?" let them know, "Why, yes, there is!"

Before you do that, though, it would be a good idea to make a list of the things that you could use some help with such as child care, food preparation, keeping up with housework, company at daily radiation treatments, rides, assistance taking care of pets, a listening ear, or maybe just quiet companionship.

*Learn to say yes, please!*

If someone is sincerely offering help, please learn to say yes! This is one of the hardest lessons I had to learn. I really struggled with letting people do nice things for me. Your friends and loved ones want to give you gifts from the heart. Please practice graciously accepting them!

I have a brother who is a researcher and a scientist, and when he offered to come to one of my first appointments to take notes, I snapped it up. And I am here to tell you, that was one of the best ideas ever. He just sat there and took notes on what the doctors said, and all I had to do was kind of take it all in. I had a list of questions to ask, and my brother asked a few questions as well. He gave me his notes after the meeting, and I referred to them numerous times when recalling what was said that day.

Having told you to say yes, please make sure that those closest to you aren't being asked to do too much and that you aren't leaning too hard on one or two people. I know, I know, that's a tough one to figure out, but cancer treatment is sometimes a fairly long haul, and you don't want to risk emotional burn-out from someone who is trying to do a good deed.

Speaking of emotions, if you have older children, I would suggest that you do not rely on them for any of the emotional heavy lifting. Don't ask your children to help process your incredibly difficult emotions when they are very likely struggling to figure this all out for themselves. Of course, I'm not saying that your kids can't handle tears or honest discussions about what's happening. That's the stinking reality of the thing, but please save the really heavy-duty stuff for your closest girlfriends or the therapist.

Finally, if, by some chance, you are in a new city or don't have a support network of friends and family to help you, please tell your doctor or nurse. She will be more than happy to connect you with a social worker who can help you figure all of this out.

The main thing to know is this: No matter the source of the comfort and assistance, you do not have to be alone on your journey through these physically difficult and emotionally exhausting times.

## THE BOTTOM LINE

Build a team, as large or as small as you see fit, and allow them to be there for you as you move through the tough days that are surely coming. You will be glad that you did. If someone wants to help you, please learn to say YES!

# 6. GET ORGANIZED

One of the many things I wish I had known at the time I was diagnosed was the critical importance of collecting, organizing, and maintaining all of the medical records (and other non-medical paperwork) that I needed to have access to on a regular basis. This is known as a Personal Health Record (PHR), and while most people don't take the time to pull all of this information together into one handy location, I swear that it will pay off handsomely if you do.

Treatment for a disease as complicated as breast cancer will entail the services of an often dizzying array of medical professionals and organizations, each holding just a small piece of the puzzle that is your medical and cancer history.

You also have a non-cancer medical history that may need to be taken into account as treatment progresses. Do you remember the results of the menopausal hormone tests that were run three years ago? What was the date of your hysterectomy? What is your blood type? When was your last electrocardiogram?

The sooner you are able to quickly and confidently retrieve all pertinent medical information, the better. I almost always carry my PHR with me to medical appointments, especially when I have an appointment in a new office. They are always surprised, and often delighted, that I can answer questions about dates, results, and treatments, all by opening my little three-ring binder and looking behind the appropriate tab.

There are a few other really important reasons to collect this information. First, when I am in a medical office, speaking to the doctor, I do not have time right that very second to look over papers and test results just handed to me, but I surely do take that time when I am sitting comfortably in my own home.

Also, as the mother of two daughters, I desperately want them to have the details of my breast cancer history available so that they too can be proactive about their breast health, if it ever becomes necessary.

Before I go any further, I really ought to confess that I am a spice alphabetizer, so this next thing is right up my alley. You may never take the organization of your records to the heights that I did, but the very best advice I can give you is to get some sort of a system set up as soon as possible—a system that allows you to have information in an easily accessible and portable location. Setting up and keeping this system organized might be one way for a support team member to help you out.

Here's the information that you *may* wish to collect as part of your PHR. You decide how deep to take this thing.

### *General medical information*

The first section of your PHR will include basic information about you, including your handwritten notes (in a medical journal that you'll start right now), your birth date, blood type, height, weight, detailed emergency contact information, allergies (including foods, animals, and medicines), vision basics, and health insurance details, including name of primary person insured, current list of immunizations and dates given, family doctor's name, address, and phone number, family medical history, a list of significant illnesses, surgeries, and treatments other than breast cancer, including childhood diseases, details of the breast cancer diagnosis (date, type, stage, etcetera), and anything else you think is pertinent. Update whenever anything changes.

I've seen many recommendations that this written (and printed out) information ought to include a social security number, but personally, *I think that carrying your social security number around is an incredibly bad idea.* I don't carry my social security card around in my wallet, so why would I keep it in my personal medical history file?

Regarding the medical journal, this is simply the dated notes that I jot down at every appointment and when talking on the telephone: Who I talked to, what was said, when it's supposed to be done, by whom, and any follow-up required. I make a neater version once I get home, and fill in any additional information while it is still fresh in my mind.

### *Your medical team*

For each doctor and nurse/nurse practitioner on your medical team, list the name, specialty, medical practice, address, phone and fax numbers (and email address if applicable). A simple and elegant way to organize this section is by collecting business cards everywhere you go and putting them in a plastic business card holder made just for your three-ring binder.

### Imaging

One of the things I know for sure is that you are going to have your breasts looked at a thousand different ways by a thousand different people (possibly an exaggeration, possibly not) as you make your way from diagnosis to survivorship, including mammograms, ultrasounds, MRIs, PET scans, CAT scans, and yes, even x-rays.

For each image that is made, it's helpful to keep track of the name, address, phone and fax numbers of the specialist and of the facility where it was made, the doctor who requested the image, the date the image was made, the type of image, and copies of all associated reports.

### Surgery

The name, address, phone and fax numbers of your surgeon and the facility where any surgery was performed, the date of each (if more than one), and a copy of the discharge summary.

### Chemotherapy

The name, address, phone and fax numbers of the oncologist and facility where chemotherapy was administered, the dates it was given, a detailed description of the treatment including type of central line, name of medication(s), dosages given, delivery method, anti-nausea medications received, and allergic or adverse reactions.

### Radiation therapy

The name, address, phone and fax numbers of the radiation oncologist and the facility where it was given, the dates it was given, the type of machine or technology used, the area treated and shielded, the amount of radiation per session, the total dose, and copies of all associated reports.

## *Complementary medicine*

The name, address, phone and fax numbers of each complementary physician or specialist, the type of medicine or therapy, the number of sessions, the date and length of each session, the symptoms treated, the side effects, if any, and any copies of any reports or assessments done by the practitioner. This would include but not be limited to occupational therapy, massage therapy, and support from nutritionists.

## *Routine lab reports, test results, and pathology reports*

This will include copies of all pathology reports, second opinions, genetic and genomic testing results, as well as lab reports, hormonal assessments, cholesterol screens, blood work panels, glucose screenings, blood pressure, and electrocardiogram reports.

## *Medications*

The names of all medications and supplements taken, both prescribed and over-the-counter, what each is for, the date prescribed, by what doctor, the dose, any adverse or allergic reactions or side effects you have experienced and changes made as a result, as well as any allergies to medications.

## *Insurance, explanation of benefits, financial records, bills, and other legal stuff*

There are a number of insurance benefits that may be triggered after a breast cancer diagnosis, including medical and hospital, disability insurance (short- and long-term), long-term care insurance, and cancer insurance.

It's a good idea to place a copy of all pages from your employee handbook that may apply in your PHR, including paid and unpaid time off, disability and Family Medical Leave Act (FMLA) benefits.

As you receive explanation of benefits (EOB) itemizations, include them in this section. Review for accuracy and make sure you include all handwritten (dated and written right on the pertinent page) notes concerning phone calls made to ask questions or straighten something out, the first and last name of the person you talked to, the number and extension, and what they said to you.

If you don't already have a copy of each of your insurance policies on hand, call the company and ask for one. They don't need to know why, and if they ask you why, you do not have to tell them.

There are a number of legal documents that you may already have prepared regarding your health care now and in the future, including a living will and a durable power of attorney. If you haven't already done so, now is a very good time to take care of these, which will give you the ability to control how you wish to be cared for in the event that things get bad, and who you want to make decisions for you if for some reason you become unable to do so for any length of time.

A living will is an especially important document, covering such topics as your wishes regarding pain management, medication, hydration, feeding, and the use of extraordinary life support measures.

If you wish to become an organ donor, this would also be a good place to include a document (or at least a statement) that will make that known as well. It should be stated here that our organ donations may be rejected in the future depending on the type of cancer, how long we were in remission at the time of the donation, and the treatments we were given.

That said, I'm still on the organ donor registry. They can figure all that out after I'm gone; I just want them to know it's all theirs if they want it.

### *Collecting and organizing this information*

It's important to note that it is unlikely you will be offered much of this information without asking for it, so please (please, please) start getting into the proactive habit of asking for a copy of everything as it is prepared, while you are actually standing in the office. This might even save a little money in the long run, as they are unlikely to charge for a copy of something that is prepared for you while you are still in the office.

Unfortunately, it will be necessary to backtrack once you realize how important this record-keeping is, depending upon how long you have been in treatment and haven't been a proactive record collector. No worries, just ask as soon as you think of it, and fill in the gaps as best you can, as soon as you can. You will probably have to pay for these back copies, but there are restrictions as to how much they can charge for this information, so it shouldn't be too expensive.

I was so thrilled about how useful it was to have all of these details at my fingertips that (once treatment was underway and I had a chance to catch my breath a little bit) I went back a few years to include all non-cancer-related medical records in the same binder.

*Free and for-a-fee computer programs*

There are also a number of companies that have appeared in the market-place, offering to put all of your health records together for you, up in the clouds, stored on a computer off-premises. These free (and sometimes for-a-fee) programs allow you to manage all of the information that I have mentioned above. You should know, however, that there is a wide-ranging debate about the security and the privacy of these systems.

There is an even more intense debate in the medical community as to how much of their own information patients should be allowed to have access to. The concern of the medical community is the same as the one that appeared with the proliferation of websites providing medical information, specifically, that people will attempt to diagnose and treat themselves.

The use of standards and regulations by online record-keeping systems is still very low. The majority of companies that design them are not covered by the stringent HIPAA laws relating to the privacy of medical information and records, which is one likely reason that these are not yet highly utilized by cancer patients.

Currently, the most popular free version is Microsoft HealthVault, which has more than 100 third-party applications available for use. The development of third-party applications that add functionality to these online systems is increasing, and, unfortunately, security issues may continue to increase as more developers enter the marketplace.

## THE BOTTOM LINE

Getting organized before you get busy (and tired) with treatment is a wise choice. Setting up a system to organize your PHR would be a great job for one of your support team members. However, be very aware of what you are putting in cloud storage and pay attention to the security design of the program if you choose this method for organizing your records.

# 7. FEED HOPE AND
# GET A GRIP ON STATISTICS

I do believe that we all have the ability to shape the general nature of our breast cancer journeys (and our lives, for that matter) by virtue of what we give the power of our attention. I'm fortunate to have been born with a generally optimistic disposition, but even that was sorely tested after my diagnosis.

One of the first women who came to walk by my side was the long-distance friend of a friend, Mary, a seven-year stage III breast cancer survivor at the time. Mary sent many words of advice and encouragement in those first months, and, as a matter of fact, her very first email included this simple yet powerful story, her adaptation of a classic tale:

*Two wolves*

A wise elder was giving counsel to a woman who was about to begin a difficult journey. "I see two wolves who will accompany you," the elder said. "They will fight with each other all along the way to determine which one will carry you through the challenges of your journey. One wolf is life-denying: Its name is Fear. The other wolf is life-affirming: Its name is Hope. The one that is stronger will be the one to carry you." The woman thought about this and then asked, "But which wolf will that be?" The wise elder simply replied, "The one you feed."

Constantly thinking about what you are afraid of, or angry about, or about how unfair cancer is, will do little more in the long-run than increase the size and strength of thoughts that serve only to move you closer to other negative thoughts. Focus constantly on the unfairness of cancer, and you will most certainly find ways to prove over and over again that this is true.

By the exact same reasoning, if you lovingly give your attention to positive thoughts, you will soon reap the immense benefit of the blossoming of hope. My dear ones, of course we will have moments of fear, frustration, confusion, and anger. The difference between allowing these thoughts to be a constant presence or simply listening to what they have to tell us and moving quietly on will mean the difference between a journey of despair and a journey of hope.

### Choose a journey of hope

So make a choice—no, a series of choices—that yours will be a positive journey, that you will actively change the nature of the chemicals produced on a cellular level. As we saw in the discussion about breathing, our bodies want very much to support us in the things we are thinking and the feelings that dominate our minds. Why not ask it to support thoughts of calm, and peace, and hope?

"But, Christine, it's so hard to be hopeful! I've read the statistics on breast cancer!" To this, I would respond that doctors do their level best to pretty much keep us away from statistics and percentages, and, generally speaking, with good reason. They can be difficult to understand. They can be complicated. And they can be scary. Most of us have had absolutely no training in how to understand them properly.

### Putting statistics into perspective

How many of us even know the difference between a mean, a median, and a mode? Remember this: Statistics are just statistics! They are neither *your* treatment nor *your* exact diagnosis nor *your* body that you are working diligently to maintain as cancer-free as humanly possible. I want you to remember that you are one-of-a-kind, and the only statistic that contains your personal, one-of-a-kind outcome is yet to be determined. And you have something to add to the calculations, something to add to the discussion about how this is all going to turn out.

You are going to run across all kinds of information in the next months and years, all relating to breast cancer and its treatment: What causes it, what might cure it, what strides have been made, alternative treatments and theories galore. You're going to read a lot of that in this book you hold in your hands. When reading about the next big thing in cancer research, especially treatments that make a big splash in popular media, ask the following questions: How big was the study? Who funded it? Were the results peer-reviewed? Were the results ever duplicated anywhere else? If you are looking at a 30-person study that took place twenty years ago that touted kumquats as a cure for breast cancer, and it was funded by the KCB (The Kumquat Council of Brazil), I think you might view those numbers just a little suspiciously.

## THE BOTTOM LINE

So here is my takeaway on statistics: Let them speak to you in a general way. Pull wisdom from them. Use them to shine light in dark corners. Use them to educate yourself, to get yourself walking on the path you wish to take, to guide your steps in the next months and years. Never use them against yourself or as a tool of judgment and negativity. And, as my friend Mary reminds me whenever she gets the chance, always, always, always remember to feed hope.

# 8. HIRE BREAST CANCER SPECIALISTS

One of my first exhortations to you at the beginning of this book was to put yourself in charge of this project, and I truly hope that you are at least beginning to wrap your head around that concept. I would be even more delighted if I knew that you had already embraced it enthusiastically! One way to take charge of your journey is in regard to your medical team.

Your oncologist is going to be a part of your life for many years to come. This primary relationship must work well for you, or you must change it. Numerous friends and acquaintances have mentioned to me that having a solid doctor-patient relationship had a decided impact for the better on their ongoing breast cancer treatment.

Until very recently, we had a medical system that was built around the idea that the doctor (probably a dude) was the infallible boss and complete authority figure, directing medical care with little (or no) input from the actual patients (especially if the patients, like us, were not dudes). We are making progress, shifting from this outdated way of doing medical business to one in which the doctor is now seen as a highly-paid consultant and expert in the area of which you have hired her.

*Every decision we make is guided by information given by the doctors*

You will count on the information and advice your doctors provide. It must be up-to-date information on your kind of breast cancer because, without that, it will be more difficult to make completely informed decisions about care and treatment.

By "your kind of breast cancer," I mean not just finding a breast cancer specialist, but also finding a doctor who specializes in your specific kind of breast cancer. It is worth the trouble to at least find out if it's a possibility.

For me, this adds up to one thing: A breast cancer patient should be giving her business to breast cancer specialists, in as many areas of medical practice as she will be encountering.

You may have a wonderful general practitioner you have loved for years and years, and a great working relationship with the entire practice, but when it comes to something this monumental, this crucial, you must pick a doctor that is specifically paying attention every single day to everything that is happening in the fast-paced world of breast cancer treatment and advancements.

### *Troubling statistics*

A study presented at the annual meeting of the American Society of Clinical Oncology, in May 2012, found that just over half of general practice doctors could identify heart problems as a possible late-occurring effect of the commonly-used chemotherapy drug, Adriamycin. Even more troubling, only a quarter were able to identify possible nerve damage to arms and legs as a result of using the cancer drugs, Taxol and Eloxatin, also commonly prescribed, and even fewer knew that early menopause and second cancers were a possible side effect of one other drug, Cytotoxin.

Now, I don't know about you, but I want my cancer doctor to be fully aware of everything related to my cancer treatment. Of course, I still see my primary care physician and he is aware of all the treatment I've undergone. I have sent him copies of all labs, reports, results, and imaging . . . but I do not get the latest and greatest breast cancer-specific information from him.

Here are some of the medical professionals that you will encounter:

### *Oncologist*

Depending upon the size of the practice your doctor belongs to, it is quite possible that you will have more than one oncologist on your medical team. If so, the primary oncologist will oversee your care in a general way, and your breast oncologist will be the doctor you will see at most of your appointments.

This is the doctor who coordinates all of your care and who you will speak to about all aspects of treatment from beginning to end. This is the doctor who you will need to have conversations with regarding all of the ways you want to approach your treatment, and this is the doctor with whom you must have the most philosophical agreement.

For me, this means that my breast oncologist is a female. This isn't to say that a male doctor isn't capable, but I do want this particular doctor to have a deeper understanding of me as a patient and as a human being, and in this specific instance, it means that I almost exclusively have chosen to work with women, if there is a choice. If it is possible, get girls to work on the girls, girls.

### Surgeon

Once again, any doctor cutting into me is going to be a surgeon who specializes in breast cancer surgery. This is an especially fast-paced field of technological advancement; I hope you will decide that your surgery will be performed by a doctor who keeps up with new techniques in breast-conserving surgery and has lots of experience removing breast cancer tumors as cleanly as possible while leaving your body with the tiniest and fewest incisions possible, whether you're to undergo a full mastectomy or simple breast-conserving partial mastectomy . . . and gets it all the first time!

### Radiation oncologist

This is the specialist who makes calculations for the dosage of radiation you are going to receive and oversees your radiation treatment. You will also have other people care for you while in this phase of treatment, including technicians, nurses, and social workers.

### Nurse navigator

In times of increasing complexity of treatment for all kinds of cancer and for patients who are becoming more knowledgeable and empowered in their decisions, most practices will assign a specific nurse to you who will be your go-to person through all phases of treatment.

### Geneticist

It is possible that the practice you have chosen will have a geneticist on staff to sit down with you and have a conversation on this particular topic, taking all of the information that is known into account, and talking to you about The Odds. If you are lucky, you will even have insurance that will pay for it.

That said, you will soon see that our genetic makeup plays a minimal role in determining whether one woman gets cancer and another doesn't, so if you don't get to speak to a geneticist, it's not the end of the world . . . and frankly, at this stage of the game, it's kind of a moot point, isn't it?

*Nutritionist*

The approach that is discussed and described in this book is based on a scientifically-proven and extremely sound nutritional and whole-cloth approach to life after breast cancer. I happen to be extremely fortunate that my primary oncologist believes in the value of nutrition as a key aspect of my treatment, but if she did not, I would seek out a medical practice that did have a nutritionist on-staff, and a nutritionist who understands how powerfully we are affected by the food that we put in our mouths.

*Naturopathic doctor (ND)*

Combining the essential wisdom of Momma Nature with the rigorous training of modern medical science, a ND will support you as you focus on holistic, synergistic, and proactive treatment techniques, helping to create a healthy environment for healing by turning to your body's built-in ability to restore health. A ND's training is built upon a foundation of classic, traditional medicine, often more eastern in philosophy.

*Complementary practitioners and social workers*

You may also wish to add other professionals to your medical team, including a chiropractor, a massage therapist, a physical therapist, a psychologist, or other mind-body professionals. Most oncology practices will also have a social worker on staff, who will guide you through services available to you as you negotiate treatment and recovery.

## THE BOTTOM LINE

It's all about what *we* need. Each of the medical and complementary professionals we select for our teams must be as open and honest as possible with us about our treatment, our outcomes, and the limits of what they know for sure.

They must have the ability to listen to us, to speak in a way that we clearly understand (using words that we understand), to ask open-ended questions that encourage us to speak, and to treat us as individuals. And please, please, please, especially for the primary doctors that will be working with you for years and years to come, make sure that they are breast cancer specialists. There's simply too much at stake.

# 9. UNDERSTAND THE BASICS
# OF BREAST CANCER

Just like every other organ of the human anatomy, our normal, healthy breasts are made up of normal, healthy cells that organize to become normal, healthy tissue that performs a number of important functions, which in this case includes milk production, structural support, blood transportation, and lymphatic drainage.

*Breast physiology*

The breasts are a system of mammary tissue whose primary evolutionary function is to manufacture milk. Tiny milk lobules group together to form lobes, and the milk is delivered via milk ducts, typically between six to nine per nipple. Underlying, running through, and supporting this system is breast connective tissue, consisting of fatty tissue (about a third of the breast) and muscle. The pectoral muscle supports the entire breast structure on the chest wall. It is somewhere in this mammary tissue that breast cancer first makes itself at home.

There is a system of vascular tissue that carries nutrients, oxygen, and glucose to the breast. Lymphatic tissue works to provide transportation to lymph fluid and immune cells, whose job is to irrigate and remove cellular waste from the breast. This system also works to cleanse the breast area of bacterial infection, viruses, and cancer cells.

Lymphatic vessels drain this waste fluid to a large system of lymph nodes, which is the reason that lymph nodes are a common site of early cancer metastasis. The axillary nodes are the nodes that get the waste first. That's why surgeons check these first during surgery to remove the tumor: If there has been a spread of cancer, it will typically be in evidence here.

*Types of breast cancer and traditional staging*

*Ductal Carcinoma in Situ (DCIS)* is breast cancer at its very earliest stage. It is confined to the milk ducts and has not invaded nearby breast tissue. *Lobular Carcinoma in Situ (LCIS)* is in the lobes. While this is not cancer, it is a pre-cancerous condition that dramatically increases the risk.

*Invasive (or Infiltrating) Ductal Carcinoma (IDC)* is the next stage of breast cancer, which has burst out of the confines of the milk ducts and has begun its invasion of nearby fatty tissue, spreading from the primary (or original) tumor. IDC is the most common type of breast cancer.

*Invasive (or Infiltrating) Lobular Carcinoma (ILC)* originated in the milk lobes and has invaded nearby fatty tissue. ILC is frequently found in multiple sites and can be difficult to detect either by examination or by mammogram.

There are other types of breast cancer, including inflammatory, medullary, mucinous, papillary, squamous cell, cribriform, tubular, and Paget's disease. You will soon realize that breast cancer is hundreds, if not thousands, of different cancers, with unique genetic-genomic fingerprints and attributes. The purpose of this book is not to go into medical detail about all of these types of breast cancer but more to reinforce the idea that there are a wide variety of possibilities.

Your oncology team is likely to have a pretty good idea of the stage of your cancer very early on, but it is not until the tumor has actually been removed and analyzed in great detail by a pathologist that it will be confirmed. The system oncologists currently use to stage breast cancer is the T-N-M System, where "T" stands for the primary tumor, as described by its size, "N" stands for the nodes, as determined by the tumor's spread to nearby lymph nodes, and where "M" stands for metastasis to distant sites, away from the primary tumor.

Once your tumor has been examined and tested, the pathology report will include a variety of other information: The nuclear grade of the tumor, the hormone receptor status, the progesterone receptor status, indicators of biologic growth rate potential, and/or c-erb status. Please ask your doctor the questions you have about your specific cancer, and what each of these pieces of information means to you in your diagnosis and treatment.

All of this information will be considered by your oncologist in making recommendations for your treatment. It will then be used to assist you in making huge decisions that determine the course of the treatment that you choose to undergo. I know this is very confusing information, but I want to stop right here and emphasize once again that it is *you* that will be making decisions, not the doctors. This is your life, and you must make only informed decisions about all of this.

You will have access to plenty of very basic information about breast cancer and staging, so that's all I'm going to cover on that particular topic.

Please take time to become familiar with all of the particulars of your cancer as presented to you on the pathology report, and ask questions until you are satisfied.

Forward-ho to some science. Not too much. Just enough to help wrap your head around this cancer thing. I promise.

*Genes: in charge of how cells grow*

Far more interesting to me (and I hope you, too) are the scientific advances being made that promise to move breast cancer treatment to a whole new level. Through the turn of the current century, breast cancer was treated as just one disease, and I have to say honestly, not with a great deal of success.

With the work that is shining lights into the formerly dark mysteries of the human genome and the complex role of protein production in cancer growth, we are coming to a new realization: Each tumor has its own unique genetic characteristics, and thus needs to be treated in a unique way. Breast cancer is thousands of diseases, some, with little genetic resemblance to any other.

When completed findings of the Human Genome Project were released in 2003, researchers were quite surprised to discover that human DNA contains roughly 20,500 different genes in 23 chromosome pairs, a drastically smaller number than originally estimated, considering the amazing complexity of the human body.

A human genome is one complete set of DNA for one complete human being, consisting of roughly 3 billion of these chromosome pairs within the nucleus of all our cells. Each chromosome contains hundreds, or even thousands, of genes, which carry the instructions for manufacturing proteins that, essentially, perform all of the chemical and biologic functions in each of the 100 trillion cells in the average human body. The very essence of us, in all our perfection, when all is well: One complete set of blueprints for one human being, inherited from our parents.

Of these thousands of inherited genes, only 30 or so are directly associated with an increased risk of breast cancer. The most common of these hereditary breast cancer genes are the BRCA-1 and BRCA-2 genes. Contrary to popular belief, only a very small percentage (10%) of women with breast cancer carries a defective inherited gene. A majority of the cellular mutations that cause breast cancer have built up in your body over the course of a lifetime and are not predisposed mutations inherited from ancestors.

These mutations—blueprint errors, so to speak—can pile up, and pile up, and pile up, until a critical mass is reached and cells start to divide uncontrollably, refusing to die a natural cell death. This information is important: Most cancer mutations are not hereditary, but are caused by cellular mutations that stack up over the course of time.

To complicate things even more, since the completion of the Human Genome Project, it has been determined that each gene manufactures a huge number of proteins, which are responsible for how cells behave. Researchers at Carnegie Mellon, under the direction of Dr. Jonathan S. Minden, have found that a single gene can express about 5,000 to 10,000 different proteins. They found that when a cell becomes cancerous, only a small number of the total proteins actually change. The progress of breast cancer in your body depends on minute, yet highly destructive, cellular changes, directed by this errant, mutated protein production that we are only now beginning to understand.

Whatever the cause of your genetic flaws, whether handed down to you or caused by cellular damage, it is the cancer cell's inability to die a natural cell death that allows a cancer tumor to find safe haven and then to grow unchecked. As the tumor grows, it encourages new blood vessels to be created to supply the nutrients and oxygen it needs by a process referred to as angiogenesis.

> A majority of the cellular mutations that cause breast cancer have built up in your body over the course of a lifetime and are not predisposed mutations inherited from ancestors.

*Advances in understanding cancer
(but not in treating it—yet)*

It was reported in March of 2012 that a team of researchers at Memorial Sloan Kettering in New York City had concluded that whether a breast cancer gene is switched on or off is determined to a great degree by genome-wide changes in the level of methylation occurring in the DNA.

Methylation is a phenomenon, also referred to as "gene silencing," the result of which is the growth of different tissues and cell behaviors in spite of identical genetic codes. In other words, two identical genes can behave very differently in spite of the fact that there has been no change in the actual blueprint. Instead, the outer part of the gene has been changed, which plays a role in deciding whether the gene will activate, and, if so, how strong the activation will be.

These researchers discovered two types of these alterations in breast cancer cells. One showed high levels of methylation, the other, low. The high methylation group, no matter the kind or nuclear grade of breast cancer, did worse and had a poor prognosis for metastasis, and as you will soon be aware, it is not typically the primary tumor that we need to be most worried about, long-term, but its return by metastasis.

Scientists at the Washington University School of Medicine at St. Louis decoded the DNA of breast cancer tumors from 50 patients, all of whom had the most common kind of breast cancer, estrogen receptor positive, and compared them to healthy tissue samples from the same patients. They found over 1,700 genetic mutations, most of which were unique to each individual. They found the two most common mutations that were already known, as well as three previously unknown mutations found in about one in three tumors, along with 21 other rare genetic mutations that were never seen in more than two or three patients.

Here's the takeaway: Each breast cancer is unique, and treatments tailored to your specific cancer are being researched right now. It'll be at least a few years. Not especially awesome news for us, but hopefully, for our daughters, who are next in line.

*Inflammation*

Along with the fight-or-flight response discussed earlier, the inflammatory response is one of the many amazing systems our bodies have developed to ensure healing, and ultimately, survival. The crazy irony is this: Our inflammatory system has been bushwhacked by cancer and is being used quite successfully as one of the primary biological mechanisms by which it grows and thrives. Cancer is an inflammation-driven disease.

I can thank the very last teacher our little school system ever employed to give students a basic education in Latin for many of the things that led me to slinging words on a page with such enthusiasm. When we were in the seventh grade, our Latin teacher, Miss Olivia Jones, taught us something that all first-year medical students learn, the four classic symptoms of inflammation: Rubor, calor, turgor, and dolor—redness, heat, swelling, and pain.

From a tiny paper cut to a huge wound, we can see the simple healing power of inflammation in action. The heat and redness show us that the blood supply to the affected area has increased, the swelling is an indication that changes in the cell walls have taken place to allow plasma to seep into injured tissues, and pain signals the release of messenger compounds whose goal is to draw attention, healing, and defensive support.

This normal and healthy inflammatory process, then, serves its intended purpose and goes away when its job is done. These four signs of inflammation are proof that cellular nourishment and healing immune activity have been kick-started.

*Inflammation and cell proliferation*

It was a scientist by the name of Virchow, as far back as the mid-1800's, who first saw a connection between ongoing and chronic inflammation at a particular site, the proliferation of cellular activity, and cancer.

In the 1980's, another researcher, Dvorak, referred to cancerous tumors as "wounds that fail to heal," a chaotic, disorganized, unresolved inflammation gone awry. And now, a growing number of contemporary researchers are confirming that these good doctors were definitely heading in the right direction.

It seems that inflammation is a complicated and extremely precise process of hormone regulation, including prostaglandins, leukotrienes, and cytokines. Some of these hormones speed up both inflammation and cell proliferation processes, and some of them slow it down. When these two basically opposing forces are out of balance, cell proliferation takes place, and as we saw earlier, more cell division means more opportunity for mutation and, therefore, more opportunity for cancerous growth.

*Correcting the broader environment*

The findings of a research team at the Fred Hutchinson Cancer Center shines a spotlight on the absolute need to correct the "broader environment of a patient's global health and behavior" in regard to increasing breast cancer survival rates, noting that cancer cells love inflammation and will do everything in their power to spur these inflammatory processes to their best advantage. One of our primary goals as breast cancer survivors, then, might well be to reduce systemic inflammation through diet, exercise, and lifestyle changes.

## THE BOTTOM LINE

As you can see by the list on the next page, being a woman is pretty risky business. There isn't *anything* we can do about most of these risk factors. However, it is that last group over which we have at least a modicum of control, and which will be the primary focus of our proactive work.

Your goal, joining me as we stroll toward a cancer-free future, will be to do everything humanly possible to make sure that the biological home you are creating in your body is absolutely inhospitable to the growth and spread of breast cancer cells. (Yes, we can do that.)

## *RISK FACTORS FOR BREAST CANCER*

· being a woman (1 in 8 will be diagnosed by age 85)

· getting older (95% are 40 or older at diagnosis)

· genetic mutations (only 5-10% of all breast cancer)

· first-degree family history of female cancer

· dense breasts

· radiation at a young age

· lobular carcinoma in situ (7 to 10 times higher risk)

· hormonal history, including first pregnancy after 35, never being pregnant, or a long menstrual history

· history of not breastfeeding

· high bone density

· high levels of blood androgens or estrogens

· postmenopausal hormone use

· *environment, toxins, and lifestyle*

# 10. INSIST ON GENOMIC TESTING
# OF YOUR EARLY-STAGE ER+ CANCER

According to the National Cancer Institute at the National Institutes of Health, early stage (stages I and II) estrogen receptor positive breast cancer that has not metastasized to the lymph nodes will most typically be treated with surgery, followed by radiation, followed by five years of anti-hormone medication of some type.

Bear in mind, though, that it is entirely possible your cancer is extremely active though small. In the alternative, it's also quite possible that your cancer is extremely passive and complacent though on the larger end of the scale. If we knew for sure how long the cancer was germinating before it was discovered, we'd have a better idea of its aggressiveness, but since we don't have that information, further testing on the tumor is warranted.

Making the difficult decision of whether to undergo chemotherapy along with the other standard of care treatments will be made much simpler once you and the doctor know more about the behavior of your particular cancer by sending it out for genomic testing.

And yes, I meant to say genomic, and not genetic, testing. Genetics is the study of inherited genes that are passed down from generation to generation. The study of genetics also involves figuring out how new characteristics can suddenly appear as a result of genetic mutation, such as eye color. Tests for the roughly 30 genes that predispose women to breast cancer, (such as the well-known BRCA-1 and -2 genes) exist, but that is determined by genetic testing.

The DNA in our genes doesn't operate in a vacuum, however. The study of the genomic nature of your cancer considers how that gene behaves in your body, because cells are influenced by their environment. (Let's say you have a genetic predisposition to breast cancer. It is not 100% certain that you will get it. That's the cell behavior part.)

Of the approximately 20,500 genes mapped by the Human Genome Project, a company by the name of Genomic Health in San Francisco identified 250 possible genes that they thought might be associated with tumor behavior. I'm not referring to the likelihood of tumor existence (that's genetics), but of tumor behavior once it does exist (that's genomics). I already had the tumor, just like you. That is the known fact. My chances of getting one at that time were 100%, a done deal, as it were.

Enter Genomic Health. They looked at those 250 potential genes and found, after extensive clinical study, that 21 of them are strongly tied to a recurrence-free 10 year survival. Their first clinical trial validated that their OncotypeDX recurrence score successfully predicted the likelihood of distant metastasis for women with estrogen receptor positive tumors. The second trial showed that their recurrence score predicted with accuracy whether chemotherapy would benefit these same women, and the third showed that it was a strong predictor of survival at ten years.

After reading about these results on the Genomic Health website, I realized that the most helpful information I could gain access to would tell me just how serious my tumor was about wanting to come back.

After your tumor sample is sent to the lab in San Francisco, these 21 genes are analyzed as to how active they are, and the result is a score between 0 and 100. If you have a low recurrence score (between 0 and 17), it has been shown that the likelihood of recurrence is low and that chemotherapy would most likely be more risky than the benefits you might receive from it.

With an intermediate score (between 18 and 31), it is not clear whether the benefits of chemotherapy outweigh the risks of side effects, and with a recurrence score greater than 31, the cancer has a high risk of recurrence and the benefits of chemotherapy are likely to be greater than the negative consequences of the side effects.

My recurrence score was (unfortunately) in the intermediate range. I would have liked a recurrence score of zero. However, when I coupled the negative puzzle piece of a pre-existing heart defect with the positive puzzle piece of major lifestyle changes, along with everything I know about myself and what is important to me, I feel confident in my decision not to undergo chemotherapy.

Others make vastly different decisions based on what is important to them and their doctor's advice and experience. There are many stories on the Genomic Health website, and I encourage you to go there to explore others' experiences and to read more about what they do.

This test ain't cheap: The cost is about four grand at the time this book is being published. Two things. First: Get this test. Second: Figure out a way to pay for it. It's that important. If I would have had to sell my car to get this test, I would have done it. Fortunately, my insurance is among the 90% that Genomic Health says will cover this testing, including Medicare.

Other research labs are taking a similar direction, aiming to develop new testing protocols that will look at a genomic predictor of response to breast cancer treatment and survival with newly diagnosed invasive breast cancer. One such test was able to predict the long-term outcomes 92% of the time, dividing the women into two groups, one referred to as chemotherapy "responders," and the other as "non-responders."

These tests are preliminary but look exceptionally promising, and will allow doctors to avoid chemotherapy for many, many women who currently receive it needlessly in order to save the lives of a small percentage that it currently helps.

## THE BOTTOM LINE

If you have early stage (I or II), estrogen receptor positive breast cancer, ask your oncologist about OncotypeDX, and insist that your tumor sample be tested. You'll get your recurrence score and a full report from Genomic Health in a couple of weeks. With these details in hand, you and your doctor will have exceptionally valuable information that you will both use to put together a treatment plan that works for you.

# 11. ASSESS TREATMENT OPTIONS

The purpose of this chapter is to give you a general outline of the options out there and to give you a framework to use in forming questions for your medical team when making decisions about which way to go with your treatment.

This is hardly the last and most detailed information you need on this topic but rather a springboard and question-generator for further discussion with your medical team and loved ones. I turned to the National Cancer Institute at the National Institutes of Health for this very basic information, and highly recommend you do the same if you would like more details.

The really good news is that breast cancer management has evolved dramatically in the last hundred years. Up until a few years ago the strategy was to cut it all out, along with as much surrounding muscle and tissue as possible and as many lymph nodes as could be found in the general vicinity. Most of the 40 or so lymph nodes draining from the breasts are in the armpit, and until recently it was fairly common for all of them to be completely eviscerated, referred to as a complete axillary dissection.

The entire breast, as well as all of the muscle that supports it and the blood supply to it, were typically removed at the same time, and this procedure is referred to as a radical mastectomy. A relative of mine had a partial radical double mastectomy just over 30 years ago for one cancerous tumor much smaller than mine, which means they also took everything but the lymph nodes on the non-cancerous side. Over the years, she has experienced various degrees of two possible complications from this once-routine surgery, namely, lymphedema and neuropathy, which means swelling and pain . . . and nerve damage and pain.

During the last 40 years or so, research has led us to the common knowledge that breast cancer, like all cancers of the organs, is not simply a localized disease, but rather a systemic or total body disease. (And did you

51

notice that my relative's radical mastectomy story fit into that 40-year time frame? Yeah, me too. Her medical team was a competent general practitioner and a competent general surgeon. Her outcome might have been better and her chest not so much like a real battlefield had she hired breast cancer specialists.)

It should be pretty much assumed that you have circulating cancer cells in your body, as they are microscopic in nature and probably left the breast area long ago in your bloodstream. That's my assumption, anyway, and if it turns out I'm wrong, I've still given myself some excellent overall care that will pay dividends in terms of quality of life in many different ways.

Thinking developed in the late 20th century that only the most accessible (and, therefore, the most likely cancer-contaminated nodes) should be removed. Until mid-February of 2011, your surgeon knew to automatically and routinely take smaller samplings of lymph nodes, usually about 10, at the same time the breast surgery was performed, referred to as axillary sampling.

> During the last 40 years or so, research has led us to the common knowledge that breast cancer, like all cancers of the organs, is not simply a localized disease,
> but rather a systemic or total body disease.

In the last few years, doctors took this node-conserving surgery a few steps further, acknowledging that fluid draining from the breast area generally flows to one lymph node in particular in the chain of nodes, called the sentinel lymph node. Major strides in lymph node strategy have recently been made, and I believe they warrant more detailed discussion due to the tremendous and long-lasting quality of life issues involved with node removal.

Rumors about a clinical trial that would stand the world of early-stage breast cancer treatment on end circulated unofficially for months in 2010, and the news officially broke on February 8, 2011, just weeks before my surgery. A number of friends and my newspaper-clipping dad forwarded copies of press releases and articles trumpeting the findings.

For a hundred years, the gold standard of care in early stage breast cancer where cancer cells had spread to the lymph nodes was to locate as many of the lymph nodes as possible, as quickly as possible, and take 'em out.

The awful logic behind this strategy was that one cell of breast cancer, nesting sweetly in this hospitably-warm lymphatic environment, would eventually find a home somewhere else, or would just stay put, doubling in size every 25 to 1000 days, until it again would become the gnarly beast that has given you and me, and hundreds of thousands of others, entrance into this club that the beautiful Gilda Radner reminded us no one really wants to be in.

## *Ground-breaking results*

The ground-breaking study divided women into two groups. One had the gold standard, meaning all lymph nodes (a median number of 17) were stripped when cellular cancer was detected in even a single node, followed by radiation. The other group had only the cancerous sentinel node(s)—the ones that were removed for testing—taken out (a median number of just 2 nodes removed) and each was given chemotherapy, followed by radiation.

Many doctors and clinics refused to send patients to participate in the study, citing the tremendous risk the participants would take on. Well, as it turns out, the women given the new treatment had a higher survival rate than those given the standard treatment. Not a bunch, just a point or two.

But have mercy ladies, if I don't want an extra point tacked onto my survival rate, I'm not paying enough attention to how all this works. Add to that the idea that we are no longer automatically required to lose a large number of lymph nodes unnecessarily, which is a big freaking deal.

In a discussion of these results, researcher Mark Kuerer stated, however, that "these results do not apply to women who have palpable nodal disease at presentation, who have received preoperative chemotherapy, who undergo mastectomies, or who do not receive postoperative radiotherapy or partial-breast radiotherapy."

This game-changing study came out just weeks before I was to have early-stage breast cancer surgery, where I was told I had a decent chance of having cellular cancer in at least one lymph node.

At the time, I didn't really understand exactly what lymph nodes did, except for knowing that they swell up when I'm fighting an infection. As it turns out, they are extremely necessary. They drain fluids from the arms and upper chest, and when you don't have them, the fluids just, well, they just stay right where they are.

When that happens, your arm, and/or your hand, and/or your chest, swells up and starts to hurt like crazy, unless you are really proactive, or really lucky. Infections can happen, and did I mention it hurts like crazy? It can be a lifetime affliction: Between 15-70% of women who lose at least four lymph nodes will experience lymphedema.

*Best surgeon ever*

Having just received all of this new information, I wrote a nice email to my nurse navigator, asking if I could engage the surgeon in a conversation on this particular topic. I told her I thought it would be great if I could be given the lymph node-sparing surgery if I turned out to be node positive.

Within an hour she wrote me back and said she would talk to him about it. She said, "If you don't hear from him by Friday, give me a call and I'll follow up." Now that's some serious customer service there.

Two days later I was taking a run when the surgeon himself called back and left a message, that went like this (I saved it, yeah, I realize I'm a complete dork, and this is an actual quote): "Hello Christine, Dr. O. I read your note and I think it's absolutely appropriate that we would follow the direction that the National College of Surgeons study suggests and I think that you would be the perfect sort of candidate to follow its recommendation with yours being a small and estrogen receptor positive lesion. You are absolutely on target with what you are asking for. I think you are absolutely headed in the right direction here. I'll talk to you soon." This is a good man.

*Surgery day*

Skip ahead to surgery day. The radiopharmaceuticals (radioactive drugs) that had been injected into the surgical site the day before performed exactly as planned, moving through my local lymph system and lighting up the nodes. The first procedure of the day involved a tomography machine, which picked up the gamma rays then being emitted by the nodes. These are the so-called sentinel nodes I referred to earlier, the ones that cancer cells would travel to first if they were spreading.

The tomo doctor drew diagrams right on my skin of the node locations the surgeon had to choose from, but one node in particular lit up the night sky in the tiny solar system under my arm, and was marked with a great big X like a pirate map, which was the way he directed my surgeon to the sentinel node location.

There was a beautiful young nurse in the room with us, not even in her 30's, and while I waited for the doctor to come mark me up, she told me how her husband had undergone 12 surgeries in the last few years for brain cancer, and how they had recently decided to get married and have a child in spite of the fact that it now appeared that he might die soon. She said to me, "We believe that a little time together is better than none, and he wants to know that I will always have our child as a reminder of his love." Cancer's reach leaves few untouched.

Because my tumor was so small, it wouldn't have been easy to locate during surgery, so right after the lymphoscintigraphy described above, I was immediately hauled to another department for a breast localization procedure to guide the surgeon right where he needed to go. The cancerous lesion was located by ultrasound, and a needle (similar to a core biopsy needle) was inserted, which, when removed, left in place a thin wire sticking out about three inches or so, with a white flag on the end of it. "Right here, doc. Follow it to the end."

For those of you who are familiar with ice fishing, we thought it looked like a tip-up, which they then taped down in order to get just a few more mammograms for Dr. O to take into surgery. I had by this time in the process of preparing for surgery had five nipple injections, a trip in a tomo machine, a map drawn on me in permanent marker, four lidocaine shots, and one localization needle insertion, followed by an ultrasound and four mammogram images. And then . . .

Phase Two of The Great Breast Cancer Eradication Project of 2011 reached completion on February 25, 2011. Phase One primarily involved a tremendous amount of thinking about cancer, and when I wasn't wrapped up in that particular activity, I also spent some energy in Phase One gathering vast amounts of information about breast cancer and how to avoid hosting it in my personal space for any longer than I necessarily needed to.

I also fired a nurse who thought I was too smart for my own good and learned to appreciate the value of breathing slowly and deeply. The "great" part in the title of the project refers to the greatness of the project, by the way, and not the greatness of my breasts, although, in retrospect, I have to admit that after focusing so fiercely on keeping both of them (and my life), that they are pretty great after all.

As it all turned out, I would have been Dr. O's first patient to follow this new protocol if my lymph nodes had been cancerous. But they weren't. And he didn't. Once again, I found myself gratefully walking the path that others fearlessly blazed ahead of me. Fearless? The women in this study must have been scared out of their ever-loving minds, but they did it anyway, and the rest of us, taking the same path after, will reap the benefits.

To the women who bravely entered the study: Blessings to you, my sisters. I continue to stand in awe of you and the miracles you have left strewn in my path. And all I really had to do was pay attention and ask for them to be mine. But I digress. Let's get back to some treatment options. There are five different kinds of standard treatment protocols for patients with breast cancer:

*Surgery*

The new theory of breast cancer as a systemic disease led to the development of dramatically less invasive surgeries that are only recently widely available. A modified radical mastectomy preserves the muscle that supports breast tissue as well as some of the lymph nodes. These further developments mean that breast cancer surgeons perform even more breast-conserving surgeries, including lumpectomy, where only the tumor is removed, partial mastectomy, where the tumor and a limited number of lymph nodes are removed, and simple mastectomy, which is the removal of breast tissue and nothing more.

If a few lymph nodes are removed, it's then referred to as an extended simple mastectomy. An experienced, knowledgeable, and well-trained breast surgeon will take as little tissue as possible to accomplish tumor excision and will leave as much of the nipple intact as possible so that if breast reconstruction is chosen the plastic surgeon has a good place to start. It is important that you hire a surgeon who specializes in breast cancer.

### Radiation therapy

This very common treatment protocol involves using high-energy radiation to kill cancer cells, or to prevent them from growing any further. Two different kinds are employed. External uses a machine outside your body, and internal uses a radioactive substance that is, by various means, placed inside your body, near or directly inside the tumor.

### Chemotherapy

This involves the use of one or more drugs that stops cancer from growing, either by directly killing the cancer cells or by preventing them from dividing further. It can be given either orally, by injection, or intravenously.

### Hormone therapy

The female hormone estrogen makes some kinds of breast cancer grow and prior to menopause is produced primarily in the ovaries. If tests on your tumor show that the cells have places where hormones can attach to it, referred to as receptors, certain drugs can be used to either reduce the production of those hormones or to block them from working.

Treatment to stop the ovaries from working is called ovarian ablation, and could involve removal, drug therapy, or radiation. The drug Tamoxifen is often prescribed for women with estrogen receptor positive breast cancer and for those with metastatic breast cancer, which is another way of saying breast cancer that comes back, or recurs.

Therapy with a class of drugs called aromatase inhibitors is given to some postmenopausal women with hormone-dependent breast cancer. Postmenopausal women are not manufacturing estrogen in their ovaries any longer, but production does amp up in other tissue, including fat cells, and in the adrenal glands. Aromatase inhibitors decrease the amount of estrogen in the body by blocking an enzyme called aromatase from performing its job of turning androgen into estrogen.

### Targeted therapy

Often it is possible to treat breast cancer with drugs or other substances that identify and go after cancer cells but leave the healthy ones alone. Included in this class of therapy for breast cancer treatment are monoclonal antibodies and tyrosine inhibitors. PARP inhibitors are another kind of targeted therapy, used for a type of breast cancer referred to as triple-negative.

### Risks and side effects

There are risks and side effects to each of these treatments. Some are easy to deal with and will disappear once treatment is done, some are quality of life issues, and some are potentially life-threatening, or at least game-changing. It's all a really big deal, but I'm not going to go through all of the possibilities here, because these are topics you must discuss with your doctor.

Ask your doctor about the side effects of the treatment(s) under consideration. Insist on the full story, and then figure out how to best handle it.

Side effects may last for many years. Advances in treatment options mean that there is a larger population of survivors than ever before. Australian researchers followed 287 survivors for a median 6.6 years, reporting that the percentage of women experiencing at least one side effect from their treatment remained stable during that period of time.

Side effects included postsurgical issues including infection and heavy scarring, skin or tissue reaction to radiation, upper body symptoms, including disability of the arms, shoulders, and hands, such as tingling and weakness, lymphedema, weight gain of 10% or more, and reduction in upper-body function.

Although prevalence decreased over time, 60% of the women observed one or more of these side effects at six years and 20% reported two or more in that same period. In this group, weight gain was the most prevalent adverse treatment effect.

Researcher Kathryn Schmidt at the University of Pennsylvania noted,

"We can no longer pretend that the side effects of breast cancer treatment end after patients finish active treatment. The scope of these complications is shocking and upsetting, but a ready solution for many of them already exists in rehabilitative exercise."

## THE BOTTOM LINE

At this stage of our treatment, we are reminded once again, sisters, of how important it is to remain aware and proactive in planning all aspects of our care, and further, in demanding that our long-term needs for rehabilitation are met by the medical community.

Whether we are talking about diminished sexual function, lymphedema, heart issues, radiation-induced lung problems, or any of the other possible short- and long-term side effects of treatment, our voice must be heard and our needs attended to. Our part of the equation is that we do everything we can to understand the possibilities and to do everything in our power to have strong, healthy bodies; theirs, to listen and respond.

# 12. COME PREPARED WITH HIGH-QUALITY QUESTIONS

Hearing the words, "You have breast cancer," is enough to send your mind reeling in a million different directions. If you are anything like I was in that moment, you might have a little knowledge of cancer in general, scant knowledge about breast cancer in particular, and, almost certainly, no knowledge about your specific subtype of breast cancer.

It's time to change that. It's time to get an education, and the best place to start is with your oncology team.

The question is: How on earth do you accomplish this in a busy medical practice and with only a limited amount of time allotted for you each time you visit?

The answer is: Come prepared. Even now I maintain a list entitled, "Questions for the Doctor." I keep this list in my planner, adding to it as questions pop into my head, often spurred by something I'm reading or when a friend mentions something that I think is an interesting piece of information. At first, this list will be really, really long. The good news is that as time goes by the list gets shorter and you will likely be asking more specific questions.

I encourage you to make the questions fit your specific diagnosis. I also quickly found out that if I left space after the question, I could jot the doctor's answer down right on the same piece of paper. I was able to recall much more information this way, and I would ask that you give it a try.

Here are a few ideas to get you started on the important task of generating your own "Questions for the Doctor" list.

1.) Exactly what kind of cancer do I have?
2.) What is your experience with this kind of cancer?

3.) What stage is my cancer, and what does that mean in regard to my treatment?

4.) Can you explain the treatments that you are recommending?

5.) What are the chances that the treatments will work?

6.) What can I expect from each of the treatments?

7.) What is the time frame for each treatment?

8.) What are the possible short-term side effects of each?

9.) What about long-term side-effects?

10.) Do you actively integrate nutrition into your treatment? How will you support me in this regard? Is there a nutritionist associated with this practice? A naturopath?

11.) If I have a question and I'm at home, who do I call? Is there an after-hours contact number?

12.) If I leave a message, how soon will my call be returned, and by whom?

13.) How much will this cost, and how am I going to pay for it?

14.) Are there any clinical trials that I might qualify for? How do I go about finding out if I qualify?

15.) Are you going to test my tumor to find out more about its makeup and behavior?

I also ran across a website that might help you formulate good-quality questions to add to the list. The site, www.QN2A.org, was designed as an interactive website where patients and caregivers can go to present questions about their cancer, its treatment and side effects, as well as many other issues surrounding their diagnosis.

Just like this book, the idea of the website is not necessarily to give you answers, but to spark you to create a set of questions perfectly suited to you and your situation.

In the beginning, take someone from your support team with you to appointments who can take good notes. Recruit your most scientific/least emotional friend or relative for this brief task. Please don't ask your husband, your children, or your best friend to do it!


## THE BOTTOM LINE

I have found through the years that I am often at my most vulnerable when in a doctor's office, and I believe this vulnerability multiplied as I became a breast cancer patient. We must learn to speak freely and honestly on topics that can, at times, be excruciatingly personal, and about private and very intimate parts of our bodies that we may not be perfectly comfortable talking about. It's for this reason that it's best to be prepared, and to have a support person along, especially at first.

# 13. GET A SECOND OPINION: IT'S STANDARD PRACTICE

There are a metric ton of reasons to get a second opinion and they all directly relate straight back to quality of medical care. You are getting ready to make huge decisions that will have a major impact on the rest of your life. They will change the trajectory of everything that happens next, and most of the choices can't be undone. You must be confident that they are based on the best medical science out there for your exact subtype of breast cancer, taking all of the current science into account.

I know that the first few weeks after my initial diagnosis were a shock-induced blur: A surprised fog hung itself between my ears. While I recall the emotions of those days in vivid detail, it is sometimes only by virtue of having kept a journal that I can actively recall the day-to-day events of my life at that time.

The likelihood of being in such a fog, coupled with the inherent fear surrounding a cancer diagnosis, doesn't make the early weeks a great time to make final decisions about the medical team you will be spending so much time with and who will have such tremendous impact on your life.

Get a second opinion from a doctor of your own choosing, one referred to you by a friend if at all possible. I'm thinking it best that you choose your own, not relying on a second opinion from a doctor who has a close working relationship with the original. (In other words, don't get a recommendation from your oncologist.)

Even better, especially for more complicated cancers, I would choose a research hospital or major cancer center, even if it means traveling a little. There is at least one that has a working relationship with several insurance providers in order to cover your travel expenses every time you go, including the clinic I travel to, Cancer Treatment Centers of America, in Chicago.

One great resource in that regard is the RA Bloch Cancer Foundation, a non-profit organization that maintains a list of multidisciplinary second opinion centers throughout the country.

## THE BOTTOM LINE

Few doctors will resent the knowledge that you are seeking a second opinion. If one did object, that would not bode well for my continued medical relationship with that doctor. In this day and age, many will even encourage second opinions to support the plan under consideration.

The good ones will have no fear of the quality-control aspect this brings to your case and the really exceptional ones will genuinely appreciate that you are looking for additional perspective on the options they are presenting to you. I especially encourage you to get a second opinion if you live in a small or rural town, if your cancer is advanced, or if your doctor has told you that there is little hope.

# 14. EVALUATE YOUR STANCE ON WORKING

Should you focus on "rest" or "normalcy"? You will have to decide for yourself. I love working, always have, and I imagine always will. A little poem by Angela Morgan sums up my general position on the topic: "Thank god for the swing of it, the clamoring ring of it, passion of labor daily hurled, at the mighty anvils of the world."

I really do find great pleasure in a strenuous workout, in yard work, and in all physical and mental challenges in general, including those found in my profession, working with juvenile delinquents. I don't work in a foundry, as suggested by the poem, but when an angry teenager decides to lose control, I'm a part of the team that must de-escalate or step in to physically manage the situation to a safe conclusion for everyone. Not participating is not an option.

Because of this attitude, my friends and family were a little surprised that I decided not to go back to work after recovering from surgery, during the seven weeks of radiation treatment. I did change oncologists when my old one (who, incidentally, wore a "What Would Jesus Do?" bracelet) decided that I needed to work full-time at this high-energy full-time job requiring emotionally and physically action-packed 12-hour weekend shifts (when other people would be able to take advantage of two days off from radiation to rest up and relax a bit), prepare for an impending move, spend time with my parents, meditate, exercise, rest, and learn everything there is to know about breast cancer and how to never have it ever again, *and* have 33 daily radiation treatments in a location 35 minutes from my home. Whew.

Frankly, if Jesus had been in on the decision-making, I firmly believe he would have wanted me to have a little rest somewhere in this brutal schedule. By the way, my new doctor felt the same way on this topic of particular importance to me.

There are many things that will come into play as you make decisions about whether, and how, to work through treatment: What you do for a living, your company's culture and policies, your relationship with your boss, your treatment schedule, how powerfully the side effects hit you and how they may affect job performance, and how important it is to you, both emotionally and financially, to keep on working.

I've known women with fairly flexible schedules and desk jobs who worked right through treatment not uttering a word to their employers that they were even ill, and were content with that choice. I also have a friend who *appeared* to sail right through treatment while working full-time, and told me that if she had it to do over again, she would have fought to stay home and focus more on self-care and emotional health, as I did.

## The ADA and FMLA

Speaking of keeping quiet about your diagnosis, the only time you are absolutely *required* to tell your employer about what's going on is if you want to benefit from the provisions of the Americans with Disabilities Act (ADA) or the Family and Medical Leave Act (FMLA).

The ADA is a guarantee that your employer must provide "reasonable" job accommodations or other adjustments that make it possible for you to work, including telecommuting, flex-time, or a lateral position, if it can be managed. You do have to ask for an accommodation and show medical proof that it's necessary.

FMLA guarantees that you can keep your job (and benefits, like the insurances that will help pay for your treatment) over a maximum of 12 weeks while unable to perform your duties for a variety of reasons, including serious health problems.

FMLA does not guarantee that you will be paid a wage, only that your job, or one similar, is there for you when you come back. You can use it all at once, or in smaller increments, as long as in the previous 52 weeks, no more than 12 weeks was used.

## Short- and long-term disability coverage

Another option is to exercise short-term or long-term disability insurance coverage, which typically will cover something like 60-70% of your full-time pay while off work. Exercising my disability policy gave me a few extra months to heal without stress or concern for the financial needs of my family.

*What's important to you? What are your responsibilities?*

One of the biggest considerations for me was simply how I felt about it, and the same may be true for you. Work can be a huge stressor, during trying times especially, and our ability to relax may be stretched thin if we have to keep up with absolutely everything. In the exact opposite way, you may consider your work to be a place of comfort and regularity and your co-workers a positive support system.

If physical accommodations are necessary and made, you very well may want the sense of normalcy and balance provided by the act of going in to work every day. Your doctors may have an opinion on this topic as well, especially if treatment leaves your immune system in a weakened state, and if your job, like mine, involves children, large numbers of people, or other possible sources of infection.

It's vital for you to honestly assess your responsibilities both at home and at work. If working is either an emotional or financial priority for you, make sure to trim other responsibilities so that you can remain calm and focused during treatment. Make sure you have an honest discussion with your oncology team regarding the likely side effects of your particular treatment. Your doctor may be able to help out by minimizing side effects and scheduling treatments in creative ways.

### *"How the hell am I gonna pay for all this?"*

As if it wasn't enough work running around getting treated for a life-threatening illness and doing your level best to stay cool, calm, and collected (and organized, too, right?), you might just be wondering how in the wide world you are going to pay for all of this. (Unless money just isn't an object, and I know few who might qualify for that brand of awesomeness.)

I hope that insurance of some kind will pay for most of it (thank you, Mr. Obama), but even with that, there will likely be co-pays, deductibles, durable goods, medications that aren't covered, and household expenses. Enlist the help of the social worker at your clinic if you need to. That's what they get paid to do!

### *Start here*

A good place to start is with agencies that provide free or discounted care to women who meet eligibility requirements, including the National Cancer Institute, American Cancer Society, CancerCare, Hill-Burton Free or Reduced-Cost Care, LIVESTRONG SurvivorCare, Medicaid, Medicare, the Social Security Administration, and the US Department of Veterans Affairs.

You will also want to check out the Patient Advocate Foundation's National Financial Resources Guidebook for Patients: A State-by-State Directory, and the American Cancer Society's state-by-state resource database that generates possible programs based on your zip code.

### Other organizations

Many other organizations that offer general financial assistance to women dealing with breast cancer include Susan B. Komen for the Cure, American Breast Cancer Foundation, KS Inflammatory Breast Cancer Foundation, and My Hope Chest Foundation. The Linking A.R.M.S. Program provides limited assistance for hormonal and oral chemo, pain and anti-nausea meds, lymphedema supplies, and prostheses. Living Beyond Breast Cancer looks to help the newly diagnosed, young women, women with advanced breast cancer, women at high risk, and African American and Latina women.

The National Lymphedema Network may help with appliances, compression sleeves/stockings, and alternative garments. Sisters Network, Inc. has a breast cancer assistance program (called B-CAP) that provides assistance for women facing financial challenges after diagnosis, including mammograms, co-pays, office visits, prescriptions, and medically-related travel and lodging expenses.

### Transportation and temporary housing

Transportation and temporary housing for you and your caregivers can be a problem, especially if the clinic that suits your specific needs isn't in your neighborhood. There are a number of programs to assist you, including Air Charity Network, Corporate Angel Network, National Patient Travel Center, American Cancer Society's Road to Recovery, Joe's House, Hope Lodges, Eldercare Locator, and Ronald McDonald House. Many out-of-state clinics, including the Cancer Treatment Centers of America, have transportation coordination departments and may provide free or reduced airfare, train costs, or mileage reimbursement.

### Fertility preservation

Fertility preservation may be an issue if you are young enough to want to keep the door open to having children. Treatments for cancer can be an obstacle and Livestrong's Sharing Hope teams up with fertility centers to provide assistance to women whose therapy presents the risk of infertility.

*Prescription assistance programs*

Prescription assistance programs provide free or low-cost medications, including the Patient Access Network, the Partnership for Prescription Assistance, NeedyMeds, Managed RX, CancerCare Patient Assistance Foundation, NORD, Patient Services Incorporated, and RxAssist. All major pharmaceutical companies have programs in place to assist patients in obtaining the specific medication they require.

Also, the National Comprehensive Cancer Network maintains an online prescription reimbursement resource room that will provide a wealth of information. If you are enrolled in Medicare Part D, you may be eligible for assistance through GSK Commitment to Access or Lilly TruAssist.

*Co-pay assistance*

Co-pay assistance may be available through the Patient Advocate Foundation's Co-Pay Relief program if you are insured and qualify both financially and medically. This agency is a non-profit with a mission to provide case management services to people with chronic or debilitating diseases. Not only does this organization connect you with others that can provide assistance, but they can help directly with insurance questions and claims appeals.

*If a claim for care has been denied*

If your first claim for care has been denied that you believe should have been covered, do not take "no" for an answer! Put your claim in until they approve it—I heard from several girlfriends that three times is the charm—and check out advice from the Kaiser Family Foundation and the Patient Advocate Foundation on how to accomplish that feat. These two organizations also have how-to's on cashing in an insurance policy to cover medical costs.

*Crowdfunding*

Crowdfunding is available if you really, really want to step outside the box. Sources for crowdfunding include YouCaring.com, GiveForward.com, GoFundMe.com, Fundly.com, and Indiegogo.com. They will direct you through the process of setting up an account, using social media and email contacts as starting points. I used GoFundMe in 2013 when I collected money for the local Gilda's Club while training for my first real half-marathon and was happy to reach my fundraising goal very quickly.

*Paying for the genomic analysis of your tumor*

Genomic Health (the company I referred to earlier that performs genomic testing on breast cancer tumors) provides financial assistance and even has a staffer who works with your insurance company to make sure the claim gets paid. They also will set up a payment plan if all else fails. Whatever else you decide to do, make sure to have your genomic analysis done. Have I impressed this on you yet? Do whatever it takes to get this testing done.

## THE BOTTOM LINE

Make sure that you demand the care you need, no matter what the expense, and then start shaking the trees for how to pay for whatever is not covered by insurance. As in all other areas of your treatment plan, you do have options.

You gotta get on the internet, or on the telephone, and start making connections. This might be a great area for one of your support people to take charge of for you, especially if she is comfortable on the telephone, is particularly assertive, and/or is adept at a keyboard.

Updated contact information for
each of the agencies discussed in this chapter,
and more, will be found at:

www.ultimatesurvivorship.com/resources

# 15. REFLECT IN SOLITUDE
# AND MAKE CONFIDENT DECISIONS

You've done the research. You've gone over and over the options and the ramifications of each. You've discussed it in detail with the major stakeholders in your life and with other women in your shoes, if you felt that was appropriate. Have all of your questions been answered? Do you have sufficient information from reliable sources?

### Pros and cons

If the answers to those two questions are "yes," then it is time to move forward in the decision-making process. There is one final way to more thoroughly assess the information that you have amassed: A good old-fashioned list of the pros and cons of each option available.

I would even go as far as prioritizing each of the pros and cons, listing them in the order of importance to you, from "this is a big deal" to "that's a consideration, but it doesn't carry much weight."

### Give the most weight to your own opinions

While taking part in all of these mental gymnastics, it might be a great time to also ask yourself if you are giving more weight to the opinions of others than you are to your own. Of course, the thoughts of our loved ones are valuable, but I can't repeat my mantra often enough: This decision is yours, and you are the one that will have to live with the consequences.

CHRISTINE ANDERSON

*Advice to your best friend*

This final reality check is one of those things that, though simple on the face of it, is exceptionally useful. If my best friend was asking me what I thought about her treatment options, and I had all of the same information available to me, what would I tell her?

This is just one more reminder that you are indeed your own best friend, and you must be just as enthusiastic and hardcore about your needs being met as you would be about hers.

*Trust your intuition and reflect*

Seriously. The finest tool at your disposal is gut instinct. Trust yourself to make these decisions. Trust yourself to know what you need to do. What is your heart telling you? What is your lifestyle, what do you hold dearest, what values are found at your absolute core?

Now is the time to sit quietly for a day or two with your thoughts. Allow yourself the time, whatever you feel is right, to reflect on all of the options available to you. You absolutely must take your time. Don't let anyone (anyone!) push you into anything *before you are ready*.

Do you have a place to go where you can briefly pull away from the rest of the world, where you can relax and quietly allow the information to wash over you? I am fortunate to have such a place, where I make all of the most important decisions of my life: I live just minutes away from Lake Michigan, where it is an easy task to find peace, quiet, solitude, and rolling waves that remind me of my place in the universe.

## THE BOTTOM LINE

All right. It's time to commit to a firm yet flexible plan. You have done everything within your considerable power to make sure that these are decisions you can live with. Now is the time to commit to a plan, confident in the knowledge that you are doing the exact thing that needs to be done, in this time, in this place, and for you.

And one last caveat: Even though this plan is the one you feel most comfortable with, please make certain that it allows for the possibility of veering in another direction, for changing your mind, if it becomes necessary.

Onward and upward. It's time to show the universe what kind of amazing star-stuff you're really made of.

# 16. DO SOMETHING YOU DON'T THINK YOU CAN DO, AND REMEMBER TO ENJOY EVERY SANDWICH

Mercy, girls, oh mercy, but the first few months of The Adventures of Christine in Cancerland were interesting, to say the least. All in all, I marched through in a blur with my sanity intact, with leaky eyes giving me trouble from time to time. This was a new and odd development. When I say leaky eyes, I mean just that: Tears that randomly leaked out of my eyes with no warning, which lasted for a few minutes and then went away.

This was most assuredly a new occurrence. I am not much of a crier, having spent a number of my formative years in a foreign tribe of generally kindhearted and stoic people who look askance at unnecessary and extreme emotional displays such as anger, passion, disappointment, sadness, and overt joy, for example.

And so, I bumped along pretty well. A support network began to develop: Visits, emails, phone calls and texts, even handwritten cards and letters. There is no real way to express adequately how much this meant to me, and the smiles they brought to my face. I am especially fortunate to have made heart-inspired connections with women who had either survived breast cancer or were going through it at the same time.

I got tremendously thoughtful and beautiful letters from two of these women right before my surgery, offering not just their personal stories of survival, but practical advice that gave me a compass for developing my own path through this often-frightening wilderness.

One of them reminded me, in the words of Warren Zevon, to enjoy every sandwich. Remember him? The excitable boy of music—Werewolves of London?—who, when diagnosed with end-stage lung cancer, decided to go ahead and put out his last album anyway, and, when asked why, in his

71

last interview with David Letterman, made the sandwich comment.

That really struck a chord in my soul at a time that I needed it most. Enjoy every sandwich! Such a brilliant and profound statement. This same woman also reminded me of a quote by Eleanor Roosevelt: "You must do the thing you think you cannot do."

I was pondering both of these thoughts as I laced up my running shoes a month into my diagnosis and headed out on a miserably cold day for a 10k run through the woods, which I have done once a week for quite a few years, with my running buddies, our dogs, Big Daddy and Bella. We moved into a quiet rhythm on the icy trail, so many thoughts of the previous weeks crashing into each other, slowly and eventually melting into the rhythmic sound of footfall on ice.

Before I knew it we were back at the house. Not feeling like I was done, Big Daddy and I left Bella at the house and headed out to run the same trail a second time. Now, I had thought of running a half-marathon before—but hadn't trained for it, wasn't prepared for it in any way, and really didn't think I could do it. Exactly how I felt about my life right at that moment.

Which is exactly why I did it.

I am not an especially fast runner, and I am most certainly not a distance runner, but it is safe to say that I was determined: It took me almost three hours to finish. In the last two miles, I began to get spasms like ice picks relentlessly stabbing my legs.

In the last mile it hurt so much and I jogged so slowly that a fast walker could easily have passed me. I wanted to stop. I was screaming inside. I pictured how wonderful it would be to just lie down in the snow, in the woods, for a few minutes. I considered calling Mike to come pick me up. I considered walking the rest of the way. It was cold, I was soaking wet. There isn't a soul in the world who would have blamed me.

We plodded ahead. And dammitall, we finished.

The spasms didn't begin to relent until I'd soaked in a deep tub filled with screaming-hot water for half an hour and did sun salutations for another half an hour. But I did something that I did not think I could do. And as I fell asleep that night, I relived my difficult run, the spasms just a memory, and I smiled to myself, and I knew in my heart that I could do the next impossible thing that lay before me.

I encourage you to do something, today, this week, that you think you cannot do. Not everyone would choose to run the Warren Zevon Enjoy Every Sandwich Almost-a-Half-Marathon, but surely there is something else, like climbing to the top of a tall tree and surveying the world from a swaying, dizzying height, or calling someone who you haven't spoken to in 10 years because you regret what you said, or holding a snake, or climbing a rock wall, or going skinny-dipping in the pool at night when you wouldn't dream of doing such a thing but have always secretly wanted to, or giving a speech, or going out to a nice restaurant all by yourself and having a perfectly delightful time. (And if you do the last one, I challenge you to do it without a book.)

## THE BOTTOM LINE

Two things: Don't forget to live, to enjoy each moment, each sandwich. And also, is there something that scares the living bejeebus out of you? Do it. Do it! Because the deepest truth is this: You can do the thing you think you cannot do. I swear to you on my honor. You can.

# PHASE TWO: THE LIFESTYLE

Nourishing,
strengthening,
detoxifying.

*"Enjoy every sandwich."*

~ Warren Zevon

# 17. TAKE CARE OF YOURSELF DURING ALL PHASES OF TREATMENT

The goal of breast cancer treatment, whether we are talking about chemo-therapy, radiation, or hormonal therapy, is to interfere with the growth of cancer cells, with the ultimate goal of destroying them. The things we need to go through in order to accomplish this will take a toll on our bodies. I started to say that they "can" take a toll, but that's not true. They will.

However, the extent of the side effects each of us experiences will be different, and will depend on the extent of the chemo and radiation used, as well as our health prior to diagnosis, along with our general approach to taking care of ourselves during treatment.

That said, there are only a couple of ways to destroy cancer cells in that big guns kind of way, and they generally involve a woman allowing herself to get her ass kicked. Because at this time in the universe of cancer treat-ment, the main way to kill cancer cells also involves killing a lot of happy, normal cells that do other wonderful and useful things for us.

There are a great number of possible side effects that you may experi-ence from chemo, radiation, surgery, and hormone therapy, including but not necessarily limited to (take a deep breath), and in no particular or-der: Lymphedema, low white cell count, low red cell count, low platelets, hair loss, hair growing in places you don't want it to, hot flashes, skin and nail changes, taste changes, mouth sores, nausea and/or vomiting, diarrhea, constipation, fatigue and weakness, disruption of sexuality, radiation-induced bronchitis or pneumonia, nerve and muscular issues, reddening or burning of the skin, weight gain, weight loss, depression, exhaustion, leg cramps, loss of sleep, and/or pain.

I'm sorry, but it's the stinking, rotten truth. The good news is that it is highly unlikely you will experience all of them. It is more likely you will experience only a few of them, depending on your treatment, and in fact, you will experience varying degrees of the ones you do get.

While you are going through active treatment, make sure you maintain proper hydration, get sufficient rest, practice breathing techniques and meditation, ask for help as needed, and exercise as much as comfortably possible.

It is vital that you keep moving to the best of your ability, especially when it comes to easing fatigue and the general malaise (and all-too-common mood depression) that often go hand-in-hand with treatment.

## THE BOTTOM LINE

This book is not about diagnosing the problems you may possibly experience or giving you specific advice on how to cope with the inevitable side effects of treatment, because that is a plan for your medical team and you to discuss and work out.

It *is* to tell you that there are lots and lots of tactics that you and your doctors can employ to successfully minimize side effects. You must ask and keep asking until you receive answers that make sense to you and fit your life.

If you have any contact with the outside world whatsoever, you are also going to get lots and lots (and lots) of advice from other survivors on things to try. I urge you to listen to your sisters, because they have been there and know what they are talking about. There are tricks and tips that can only come from the field, and they can make the difference between "relatively comfortable" and "holy wow, this really sucks."

# 18. TAKE TIME TO CELEBRATE . . . AND THEN GET READY TO CHANGE YOUR PARADIGM

If you have now completed the initial treatment for your breast cancer, it's celebration time! You've made it through a great deal (slash, burn, and poison, as one girlfriend wryly noted) and are now finally able to make plans to move forward with the rest of your life as a breast cancer survivor.

This is a definitive place, a critical place, an important juncture, a pivotal crossroads, a—well, you get what I'm saying. This is the place where you will part ways with most women who have been in our shoes. You're already a survivor, but this place, my dear sister, is where the rubber meets the metaphorical road.

The majority of women, having gone through the rigors of treatment (by whatever means or degrees this has been accomplished), look at themselves in the mirror at this point in the game and gratefully say, "Enough. I'm done. The cancer has been extracted. Treatment is now complete. It's time to get back to my *real life* and time to move on."

Some will take their meds, some, inexplicably, will not. Many women now believe that the work has been done because the cancer has been eradicated permanently.

This is not an attitude that I will choose. I do not wish to rest on the idea that my cancer will never come back, and so: I will not return to the exact same lifestyle that got me here in the first place. There is some important work yet to be done, and I view it as some of the most important work of a lifetime.

As much as I appreciate some aspects of the doctor-type television shows that help women learn to take better care of themselves, I think there is also a real danger in that their short, cute, and well-produced little segments encourage us to do "this one thing that will change everything," or to "take this one supplement (raspberry ketones, green coffee bean extract, turmeric extract, and on and on) to fix your problem forever!"

In my opinion, the truth involves much more of a commitment to overall change. I believe, for me, that what needs to happen is a synergistic, whole-life, whole-body, whole-house approach to staying cancer-free. I realize it's going to require that I make deep and honest changes in the way I go about my life's business, and further, that there won't be anything quick about it.

Study after study has shown that women diagnosed with breast cancer who make a concerted effort to stay physically active, maintain a healthy weight, and eat a well-balanced, plant-strong diet are much more likely to survive than those who don't. As early as 2002, the *Journal of Nutrition* reported that epidemiologic studies have provided links between diets high in fruits and vegetables and an increased likelihood of survival from breast cancer, and that clinical studies identify obesity as an extremely important prognosticator of recurrence.

> Study after study has shown that women diagnosed with breast cancer who make a concerted effort to stay physically active, maintain a healthy weight, and eat a well-balanced, plant-strong diet are much more likely to survive than those that don't.

In 2011, the National Academy of Sciences undertook a definitive study of the impact of various environmental factors on breast cancer, poring over a large body of evidence and issuing a massive report entitled *Breast Cancer and the Environment: A Life Course Approach.*

They defined environmental factors affecting breast cancer causation in an exceptionally broad and wide-ranging manner to include anything not directly caused by genetic inheritance.

The committee reviewed hundreds of studies on the following topics: Oral hormones and hormone therapy, body fatness and abdominal fat, adult weight gain, physical activity, dietary factors, tobacco smoke (both active and passive), radiation, shift work, metals, consumer products, industrial chemicals, pesticides, PAHs (from chemicals such as naphthalene and from food cooked at high temperatures), and dioxins. Within this definition, their focus was on any "exposure to physical and chemical toxicants, and on individual behavior related to diet and physical activity."

The committee, their task thus defined, found that the clearest evidence for environmental causes of breast cancer involved a combination of hormone therapy products, current use of oral contraceptives, overweight and obesity among postmenopausal women, alcohol consumption, and exposure to ionizing radiation.

Further, they found that greater physical activity is associated with decreased risk. They noted that some major study reviews have found that active and passive smoking can cause breast cancer, acknowledging that some describe the evidence as limited.

For several other factors reviewed by the committee, the evidence was not as strong but suggests a possible association with increased risk: Passive smoking, shift work involving night work, and the toxic (yet oddly common) chemicals benzene, 1,3-butadiene, and ethylene oxide. In the case of BPA (a plastic hardener) and other suspected carcinogens, the committee found that while human studies were not yet available or were lacking, findings led them to conclude that the connection is "plausible."

You do not need to commit to perfection, but it would be an incredible gift of self-love to commit to educating yourself, to continuous change, and to week-by-week advances in taking good care of yourself. I consider this another kind of perfection: A perfection of the art of growing older, which is, personally, my fondest desire, and which I genuinely hope you might share. This is no time for halfway or half-in. Prepare to make changes that will allow you to reap the benefits of spectacular good health.

There is a ton of really, really good news to share with you here. Not only will you be doing everything humanly possible to make sure that breast cancer doesn't feel welcome setting up shop again, but this new lifestyle you are about to embark on will also provide cardiac, diabetic, and immunological good health for the rest of your life.

While we are here, let's really rejoice in being here! Let's not sit on the couch anymore. Let's get active! Let's eat good food that nourishes our bodies and souls, and spend time with people that matter to us, and let's face each day with an attitude of joy and gratitude.

And so, this is the important place where I urge you to participate in your own health and well-being, where you will show yourself how very much you never want to have breast cancer (or any other kind of cancer, for that matter) ever again. This isn't a complicated process. In fact, this is a simplification of your life from which you will reap abundant rewards. This joy can't help but ripple out from you, like it has from me, in astounding ways. And all you have to do is this: Begin. Do as much as you can, as soon as you can, as soon as treatment is completed.


## THE BOTTOM LINE

You've made it through some pretty crappy stuff. It's time to celebrate how far you have come as only you know how to do it. And then, it's time to go all-in for making your body inhospitable to cancer ever again. Let's hit the floor running (or at least walking moderately fast).

# 19. AIM FOR A HEALTHY WEIGHT

I am fully aware that the topic of weight is littered with emotional landmines for many of us—me too, trust me—so I thought the best idea was to trot that conversation right out into the middle of the room and start talking.

I grew up in the era of Susie Orbach's *Fat is a Feminist Issue* and I was a regular subscriber to *Mother Jones* for many years. I bristle at the idea that I need to be a certain weight to please other people, or to please a society that has a morally dubious vision of what a woman needs to look like.

I think I am just the right height and build. For me. I am somewhat on the tall side, and have marched up and down the scales throughout the years, tending to be decidedly more curvy than not. These weight changes weren't the result of a quest to be society's crazy idea of what I ought to look like, but generally revolved around the health aspects of diet and exercise along with the way I was originally created.

In spite of a generally contentious and spectacularly dysfunctional relationship with my mother, she did give me a couple of awesome emotional gifts: She thought I was smart, and talented, and pretty, and just the right size. Not only did she think so, but she told me so.

She also loved to cook, and she loved veggies. No matter that the rest of the mother-daughter relationship would surely benefit from a serious stint of long-term therapizing, those are some pretty amazing takeaways for a little female in this society, I'd say.

This discussion about our weight isn't about shame or disliking our bodies or shapes, or the way you or I look; it's not about skinny, or ideal, or fat, or what society thinks. I encourage you to love yourself just exactly the way you are, today, right now, no matter your shape or size.

You and I are perfectly made versions of ourselves, and now, if all goes well, we are going to love and nourish our perfectly made bodies with a great deal of good food and exercise, because the bottom line in all of this is that women who are in the normal range for weight are not only less likely to get breast cancer (too late for us in that regard), but they are less likely to have a recurrence.

For purposes of this discussion, a woman's healthy weight will fall within a typical Body Mass Index (BMI) range of 18.5 to 24.9. Current epidemiological science concludes with confidence that a BMI of 25 or higher is directly tied to the increased progression of a number of cancers, including breast.

The actual connection between breast cancer and obesity appears to be complicated and only now are we really beginning to get a grasp on just how complicated it is. However, the consensus in the scientific community is clear: Obesity is a well-established risk for the development and recurrence of breast (and other) cancers. Ewerts *et al* found that breast cancer mortality after 30 years was increased by 38% in obese women and that these women were also more likely to die of non-cancer-related illnesses in that period.

The conventional view of adipose tissue simply as "fat storage" no longer carries weight (ha ha, a little science joke there). It has been found to be a complex, essential, and highly active metabolic and hormone-producing organ. In addition to the actual fat cells (where excess lipids are indeed stored by your body), fat tissue also contains a structure of connective tissue, along with nerve tissue, transportation cells, and immune cells.

These components work seamlessly to perform essential bodily functions. Adipose tissue not only responds to signals from traditional hormone systems and the central nervous system but also manufactures substances with important functions. Adipose tissue is also a major site for the metabolism of sex steroids and substances called glucocorticoids, which have anti-inflammatory abilities.

*Hormones and globulins*

We know that a primary factor in increased risk of hormone receptor positive breast cancer in obese women relates to the elevated level of circulating estrogens, which is related to increased adipose tissue mass and the production of aromatase, an enzyme that plays a key role in your body's production of estrogen, which feeds estrogen receptor positive breast cancer.

Obesity is associated with reduced plasma levels of globulin, a protein that binds and restricts the biologic activity of estrogens. Weight loss has been shown to increase concentrations of globulin.

## Insulin

Obesity is a cause of insulin resistance, which displays itself as high blood levels of insulin and impaired glucose tolerance, a prediabetic state. Studies have shown that high levels of fasting insulin in patients with breast cancer have been associated with distant (not in close physical proximity to the original tumor) recurrence and increased mortality.

Further, insulin has been implicated in cancer progression as a cell-division stimulator that delays cell death and assists tumors in building a blood supply. Now *that* is a triple threat to my health and well-being.

## Inflammation

Activated microphage cells in adipose tissue, which are key players in immune response, produce large amounts of substances that assist in the inflammation process. Study has also established that a subset of immune cells called invariant natural killer T cells link fat build-up with inflammatory processes. Obesity causes inflammation in adipose tissue, which could well contribute not just to insulin resistance but to the development and progression of breast cancer.

## Growth factors

Certain hormones have been shown to be overexpressed in breast cancer patients, which has been found to be linked, in theory, to a combination of overexposure of cells to insulin and insulin-like growth factors and/or hormones.

## The WHEL study

The Women's Healthy Eating and Living (WHEL) study concluded that women who ate a healthy diet, including plenty of low-fat and fiber-rich vegetables and fruits, were able to reduce their estrogen to safe levels. Adding exercise to the mix, the same women were able to reduce mortality by an additional 50%.

The *Journal of Clinical Oncology* reported recently that researchers at the Fred Hutchinson Cancer Research Center found that obese women who used a combination of diet and exercise not only decreased their weight, a key risk factor, but lowered their levels of several hormones.

Weight loss increases the concentrations of adiponectin, a substance that plays a part in regulating glucose levels as well as in fatty acid breakdown. It also causes a drop in the level of those proinflammatory substances that play a part in making your body hospitable to cancer growth.

All of the dramatic changes brought on by obesity are reversible by the simple mechanism of body weight reduction. I do understand this is a somewhat confusing message: Love yourself exactly the way you are, but lose weight that places you in the overweight to obese categories of the BMI chart. I guess the best way to explain myself is by saying that I don't think any healthy external changes can truly happen when we are internally hating-on ourselves or our bodies.

I genuinely believe that we are perfectly made just the way we are, with all of our infinite shapes and heights and colors and combinations thereof. I also believe that one way we can express love to these one-of-a-kind bodies is by giving them the nourishing food and gentle exercise they so richly deserve.

## THE BOTTOM LINE

Love yourself first and foremost, exactly the way you are, this very moment. When we combine the kindness of self-love with exceptional nourishment and gentle exercise, our days will be filled to the very brim with the good things our bodies need to assist in the healing process.

# 20. EXERCISE MODERATELY
## FOR THREE TO FIVE HOURS A WEEK

The very last thing we ought to do right now is the thing we want to do the most, which is to dive into a gigantic pile of comfy blankets in the warm nest of our beds and not emerge until the coast is clear. (No worries, this isn't completely off our list of things to do.) That said, it is vitally important that we keep our bodies moving through all phases of treatment—and beyond.

Early on, I asked my oncologist whether she thought it was okay for me to continue my running program and her response was, "Not only is it okay, it is imperative that you keep your body in motion right now. Don't exercise to exhaustion, but do something every day that increases your heart rate and strengthens your muscles, even if it's just an enthusiastic walk in the woods. Use it or lose it. This is a crucial time."

*A wide variety of benefits*

Two meta-analyses in particular conclude that there is an impressive list of benefits to exercise for breast cancer survivors, including maintaining (or even improving) body composition, weight loss, increased aerobic capacity, muscle strength, self-esteem, depression or sad mood relief, and an overall increase in general good health and immune function.

There will also be a happily-concurrent decrease in other lifestyle health issues such as cardiovascular diseases and diabetes. While there are not a huge number of studies that offer insight into the importance of exercise as an appropriate risk-reducing intervention for breast cancer survivors, they certainly do exist.

Studies assessed in several recent meta-analyses showed that positive outcomes were not necessarily tied to exercise in and of itself, but to the effect exercise had on biomarkers that are known risk factors for breast cancer, including weight, BMI, sex hormone levels, insulin and leptin levels, as well as the proper regulation of cell death. (But I'll take all that nonetheless.)

Physical activity has been linked to lower levels of circulating ovarian hormones, which likely explains a small portion of the complicated relationship between exercise and estrogen-fed cancer recurrence. In one large study, lack of activity was also associated with weight gain during treatment, which is linked to lower survival.

### The best news of all

There is a decrease in both recurrence and mortality risks for breast cancer survivors who exercise. The *Journal of Clinical Oncology* reported in 2008 that women who increased physical activity after diagnosis had a 45% lower mortality risk, while women who decreased physical activity after diagnosis had a fourfold greater risk.

A team of researchers at the US National Cancer Institute, led by Rachel Ballard-Barbash, analyzed data from 27 observational studies on a variety of cancer types and concluded that the evidence was strongest for breast cancer patients, noting that exercise significantly reduced mortality from all causes, including breast cancer. A meta-analysis performed in 2011 by Ibrahim *et al,* including 12,108 post-diagnosis women, found that moderate physical activity reduced mortality from breast cancer by 34% and reduced disease recurrence by 24%.

### But how much?

The next question that came to mind as I read and processed all of this information related to the amount and intensity of exercise necessary to achieve these results. For that, I turned to the research of Thierry Bouillet, who determined varying "doses" of exercise appropriate for different kinds of cancer.

Bouillet's found that there was a measurable effect for breast cancer survivors who exercised the equivalent of walking three to five hours each week, which, for most women, might be a do-able and reasonable amount of exercise. Please talk to your doctor about the safest way to accomplish this goal!

Further, in 2005, the *Journal of the American Medical Association* reported the same findings from the Nurses' Health Study. The researchers concluded that physical activity after a breast cancer diagnosis may very well reduce mortality rates and found that the greatest benefit occurred in women who performed the equivalent of walking three to five hours a week at an average pace.

## *Add strength training*

It was noted in a review of the literature presented in the *Journal of Aging Research* that while breast cancer is "highly treatable using hormone suppression therapy, a constellation of side effects ensue which mimic typical aging effects but at an accelerated pace."

The review concluded that it appears strength training is an effective therapy for many of these side effects including reduced muscle mass, reduced strength, reduced bone mineral density, as well as increased fat mass, insulin resistance, and fatigue.

A randomized and controlled study completed in 2011, and reported in the journal *Cancer Epidemiology, Biomarkers and Prevention*, assessed a twice-weekly strength training program for breast cancer survivors, finding that the participants increased muscle mass, decreased body fat, and decreased insulin-like growth factor.

It was further found that strength training stopped bone loss and built muscle in postmenopausal breast cancer survivors, especially relevant for women on aromatase inhibitors, who tend to lose bone mass while undergoing this common treatment.

It is widely accepted that higher levels of weight-bearing exercise are associated with weight maintenance, preservation of lean mass, and reduced body fat. Adding strength training has been found to increase these results, and I am thinking it may be just the extra bump we need to move to a higher level of health.

## *A few final thoughts*

It is important that you talk to your doctor before beginning any new exercise routine. Don't push too hard, too fast, especially if you are not already in the habit of exercising. Try a variety of exercises to see what you enjoy the most. While in treatment, it is especially important to keep the exercise safe and gentle, so keep it easy, and keep it fun.

And finally, wherever else your day takes you, get up off the couch and take a nice walk, even if that means simply a stroll around the yard for a few minutes.

I find that in the weeks I take the time to schedule my workouts and write them down in my planner, I am roughly a thousand times more likely to complete each of them. It seems that when I write it down, it becomes something that I am much less likely to ignore, either by scheduling something else that might be more fun, by just plain forgetting, or by running out of time.

## THE BOTTOM LINE

Your efforts to include exercise in your life on a regular basis will be richly rewarded, not only in overall good health and reducing recurrence percentages, but in what my precious Grandma Walthorn, who was up on a ladder and painting her house late into her 70's, would have referred to as good old-fashioned vim and vigor.

# 21. UNDERSTAND THE BASICS OF
BREAST CANCER NUTRITION

*Nutrition* quite simply refers to the synergistic and "wholistic" effects of the foods and drinks by which we nourish ourselves and the fuel that we provide for all of the intricate, complicated, and amazing tasks that our bodies are responsible for.

The understanding that nutrition affects our health and well-being is likely as old as the human species, but it wasn't until the late 1700's that we really began to study nutrients and their functions in human systems, how they can restore or impair health, provide immunity from disease, and influence the functions of the body (for better or for worse) in numerous and dramatic ways.

There are more than 50 known nutrients present in food that are known to play a part in human health, with six very broad classifications: Carbohydrates, proteins, fats, vitamins, minerals, and water. There has been a sophisticated expansion in the last few decades in the area of molecular and nutritional biology such that we are really beginning to understand nutrient-gene interactions and the possibility of manipulation of genetic expression by dietary means, that is, studies that ask the question, "Can nutrition affect the way genes behave?"

Additionally, the effects of over 12,000 different known substances in plant foods, produced by the plants for hormonal, attractant, and protective reasons, are being studied in some depth, and there is evidence that many of them offer protection against a wide range of human conditions.

The condition we are most interested in right this very second is breast cancer. There is great power in the wisdom that we have available to us. All we have to do is pay attention to current scientific inquiry to be heading in the right direction.

## *Carbohydrates*

Carbohydrates are found in a wide variety of foods, including baked goods, beans, popcorn, potatoes, pasta, and sugar. The most plentiful types of carbohydrates are starches, fiber, and sugars. Until fairly recently, nutritionists used a carbohydrate system in which carbohydrates were divided into simple and complex, or "good" and "bad" carbohydrates.

While this most certainly does stand up to nutritional science, it seems that it is a bit more complicated than that. Our digestive system does break down all carbohydrates (simple or complex) into simpler molecules, or at least tries to, and turns most of them into glucose (*aka* blood sugar), an energy source widely useable in the human body.

Simple carbs flood the system with glucose, causing system stress, and complex carbs tend to enter the system in a more orderly fashion, allowing a stable blood sugar situation to be maintained.

## *Fiber*

We do not, however, metabolize fiber, which passes through undigested. There are two kinds of fiber: Soluble, which dissolves in water, and insoluble, which (you guessed it) doesn't. While not technically a true nutrient, both are hugely beneficial to the human animal, performing several extremely important tasks, so I do want to talk about them a bit.

*Soluble* fiber grabs hold of fatty substances in the intestinal tract and ushers them out as waste, with the result of lowering LDL or "bad" cholesterol levels in the blood. It also regulates how our systems utilize sugars, with a result of moderating hunger and keeping blood sugar levels on an even keel. Soluble fiber can be found in oatmeal, oat bran, citrus fruit, and barley, among others.

*Insoluble* fiber (the one that doesn't dissolve in water—think of it as "roughage") moves food through our digestive system in an expeditious manner and is also responsible for assisting with hormone excretion. Great sources of insoluble fiber are beans, legumes, fruits, and vegetables, especially the skins.

## *The process*

When you eat carbohydrates, your body breaks them down into simple sugars, which enter the bloodstream. The pancreas is triggered to make insulin, a hormone that tells the cells that it's time to start absorbing this fuel source, either to be used, or stored. As the cells absorb it, blood sugar levels start to go back down, and the pancreas puts out a different substance, a hormone called glucagon that tells the liver to release stored sugar. This is an intricately tuned and ancient song, call and response, ensuring we have the proper fuel supplies for the tasks being performed.

When this system is broken, it has a major impact on the way our bodies function. Poor eating habits can be a major contributing factor to insulin resistance, which occurs when the cells don't open up to those pancreatic cells' call to start absorbing sugar. If left unchecked, insulin resistance will wear out the cells that make it to the extent that insulin production slows, and eventually stops altogether.

When this happens, it can contribute to a number of health crises, including high blood pressure, low HDL ("good") cholesterol, high triglycerides, and obesity, which the medical community now knows is a major consideration for breast cancer survivors. The plant-based diet recommended for breast cancer survivors focuses on high-fiber, high-nutrition whole foods that help stabilize sugar levels and assists with weight goals.

### Recommended dietary goals for carbohydrates and fiber

My nutritionist advised me that the overarching goal of breast cancer survivors in the area of carbohydrates and sugar is to eat less white bread, white potatoes, crackers, chips, processed foods, sweet treats, refined foods (which typically have the fiber removed), refined flours, high fructose corn syrup, and sweetened drinks (including fruit juices, which have no fiber whatsoever), and to replace them with whole grains, beans, sweet potatoes and vegetables, unsweetened drinks, and water.

She also said that breast cancer survivors are being advised to aim for between 35 and 40 grams of fiber a day, from whole grains, vegetables, fruits, and beans. This would translate into four to six servings of whole grains, one to two servings of beans or legumes, and nine servings of fruits and veggies a day, with an emphasis on choosing a minimum of three different colors each day for maximum nutrient values.

### Protein

Protein is a nutrient that must be obtained solely through diet. Proteins are responsible for building and repairing body tissues such as hair, bones, skin, blood, and other cellular structures. They also help antibodies fight infection and heal wounds, and play a part in hormonal and enzymatic regulation. Protein also has a role in gene and chromosome creation and repair.

Nutritionists further advise women to consume somewhere between 46 and 55 grams of protein each day, depending upon weight, build, and physical activity. An illustration of just how easy it is to get adequate plant-based protein is as follows: Whole-grain toast and peanut butter (6½ grams), six ounces of nondairy yogurt (6 grams), two tablespoons of raw almonds (4 grams), a cup of lentils (18 grams), a cup of bulgur wheat (6 grams) and a cup of cooked spinach (13 grams), for a total of 53½ grams.

This wouldn't even count the protein found in the other vegetables you would be eating on the same day. That's right, there is protein in almost all plant foods, including veggies, except for oils and some fruits.

### Fats

Fats are the most concentrated form of energy available to us at nine calories per gram, more than twice that of carbohydrates or proteins. To get a better picture of what that looks like, there are four grams of oil in a teaspoon, for a total of 36 calories. One cup of oil contains a whopping 216 grams of fat, for a ridiculously outrageous 1,944 calories, with zero fiber, vitamins, or minerals.

That's why it's advised that we use oil sparingly, although as breast cancer survivors, we do need a little olive oil in our diet. (We'll discuss why in a later chapter). We also need fat for the structure and upkeep of cells and hormones, for hair, nails, and skin, as well as the metabolism of fat-soluble vitamins, including A, D, E, and K.

As long as we are consuming enough calories, we can synthesize most of the fat required by our bodies, but we must obtain a small, balanced amount of two essential fatty acids (EFAs) from our diets, and they are vital to our health: Omega-3 and omega-6. Omega-3s come from nuts and seeds, including flaxseed, chia seed, and hemp seed, as well as olives, olive oil, and avocados. Unfortunately, the typical western diet is dangerously high in omega-6 fatty acids common in seed oil (corn, canola, and soybean), animal fat, and processed foods.

The goal is not to get more omega-3, but rather to balance it with the omega-6 in your diet. Excessive amounts of omega-6 fatty acids promote many diseases, including breast cancer, and increased levels of omega-3s exert suppressive effects.

It is recommended that fat be limited to 10-25% of daily calories.

### Vitamins and minerals

There are 13 generally recognized vitamins required by the human body, and they have a wide-ranging set of functions, including metabolism and cell growth regulation, antioxidation, and helping enzymes in their work as metabolism catalysts. All of the essential minerals and vitamins required by the human body can be found in a plant-based diet.

Bear in mind that it is extremely important for breast cancer survivors to keep tabs on possible deficiencies. Vitamin D is a common deficiency among breast cancer survivors and one that I shared upon diagnosis. Plant-strong eaters in particular are advised to pay attention to vitamins D and B12, and iron levels, eating the proper foods—including nutritional yeast, a yummy, cheesy-flavored food, beans, spinach, and fortified non-dairy milks—and supplementing as needed for deficiencies found along the way. (I live in Michigan, where, in the winter, we sometimes only see the sun for a few hours every few weeks, so I take a vitamin D supplement, and when the sun is shining, I give my mushrooms a sunbath. More on that later.)

Adult humans must include nine trace minerals in their diets, including iron and zinc. Many of the minerals we require support body cells and structures, and they work to regulate biological processes. For example, chromium keeps blood glucose at normal levels, and selenium works hand in hand with vitamin E as an antioxidant, which prevents cells from being damaged by oxygen.

*What we need in our diets*

In order to nourish our bodies in an optimal manner, we need to eat a wide variety of vegetables, making sure to include crucifers such as broccoli, cauliflower, Brussels sprouts, cabbage, and kale, as well as bok choy and radishes, each and every day (nine half-cup veggie servings total).

We need to eat freshly-ground flaxseed (one to three tablespoons a day), containing lignans, which may decrease tumor growth and stimulate cancer cell death. We need to eat beans and peas (also called legumes), which are an excellent source of fiber and phytochemicals, including coumestrol, which may help decrease the risk of hormone-positive tumors. We need to drink four small cups of green tea.

When (sparing) fats are used, we need cold-pressed olive oil and healthy fats with their nutrition content intact, from whole foods, such as nuts, seeds, and avocados. Our bodies also crave good, clean water.

The Physicians Committee for Responsible Medicine has put together the New Four Food Groups, and it translates well to the dietary needs of breast cancer survivors: Fruits, legumes, whole grains and vegetables. We will also put an emphasis on clean, fresh, organic, and pesticide-free foods.

*. . . and what we don't need*

Saturated fats, found primarily in animal products, including red meat and dairy, are not required in our diets, including butter, coconut oil, palm kernel oil, lard, full-fat dairy products and cheese, and ice cream. Processed meat, including ham, bacon, pastrami, salami, sausage, pepperoni, hot dogs, and deli meats are well worth turning our backs on forever. They are all preserved by smoking, curing, or salting, and are loaded with chemicals that are known carcinogens.

Alcohol intake is advised to be strictly limited or avoided altogether. Consumption of alcohol is associated with an increased risk of cancer recurrence; it is known to increase estrogen levels. Sugary drinks (including processed fruit juices) are a nutritional wasteland. While there may be some nutritional value in a glass of fruit juice, the fiber has been stripped out and nutritionists tell us that we might as well pop the top on a can of soda.

*Great resources for a whole foods plant-strong diet*

I've listed a ton of resources for the modern-day woman who is interested in moving toward a nutritionally-complete whole foods, plant-based diet on the website that is a companion to *Ultimate Survivorship: The Breast Cancer Manual*, at www.ultimatesurvivorship.com/resources/books.

Two of the best books on the topic of vegan nutrition for women are *Becoming Vegan* by Brenda Davis, RD, and Vesanto Melina, MS, RD, and *Vegan for Her: The Woman's Guide to Being Healthy and Fit on a Plant-Based Diet*, by Virginia Messina, MPH, RD. I encourage you to pick these two books up at the library, as they will cover the science behind a plant-based diet in far more detail than I could possibly discuss here. The information in these was so valuable to me that I purchased copies for my home library.

I have been tremendously inspired by the work of Dr. T. Colin Campbell, who has researched the negative effects of a diet based on animal protein, as well as the positive effects of a whole foods plant-based diet, for decades. His book, *The China Study*, was among the first I read as I began my research after diagnosis. It's a classic, and, further, it provides a solid foundation of evidence-based recommendations for creating our "new normal" lives after breast cancer.

## THE BOTTOM LINE

Generally speaking, the nutritional requirements of the human body are fairly simple, and can be easily met with a whole-foods, plant-based diet, including veggies, fruits, beans, legumes, whole grains, nuts, and seeds.

# 22. EAT FOUR TO SIX SERVINGS OF WHOLE GRAINS DAILY

We seem to have moved into this nutritionally weird place where carbohydrates have been demonized as unhealthy, when, in fact, they are vital to the optimal functioning of our bodies. A low-carb diet is not the answer to any health or weight concerns that breast cancer survivors have to deal with. Carbs are not the enemy, and it's unfortunate that so many of us have been brainwashed into thinking they are.

Quite the contrary, our goal is a simple one: To increase the *quality* of the carbs we eat while endeavoring to seek out and eliminate each and every processed, white flour, white rice, bland, tasteless, yucky, gross, nutritionally depleted, gigantic waste of space in our cupboards crappy food extravaganzas that we can locate anywhere in our homes, cars, and offices, and throw them all in a big nasty pile in a landfill somewhere, hopefully where there isn't any innocent wildlife that we might accidentally mess with when we do. (But how do I really feel?)

The healthiest carbohydrates are foods rich in essential nutrients, phytochemicals (which you'll hear more detail on very soon), and fiber, all powerful tools in our cancer-eradicating toolbox, including whole grains, legumes, beans, veggies, and fruits. The rest have got to go. Seriously.

Refined grains are dangerously deficient in all of the things we need from them, while whole grains are loaded with a variety of compounds responsible for vital biologic activity. They contain antioxidants, such as phenolic acids, flavonoids, and tocopherols, which are substances with weak hormonal effects, such as the beneficial lignans in flaxseed.

Whole grains are also rich in compounds that have an influence on fat metabolism, such as phytosterols and unsaturated fatty acids. You don't have to know or memorize any of the fancy names of beneficial things found in whole grains, but I do want you to remember this: All of these compounds and their biologic effects have been positively associated with reductions in cancer progression and recurrence.

Most of the cancer-protective compounds found in grains are in the germ and the bran, which are eliminated when grains are refined, rendering them nutritionally poor. Grains thus neutered are referred to as enriched, which means that a weak attempt has been made to restore nutritional content.

### *Look for these words when shopping for whole grains*

When you see the following words on a nutrition label, they will lead you to foods that contain all parts of the grain: Whole grain [grain name], whole [grain name], stone-ground whole [grain name], brown rice, oats, oatmeal, wheat berries, and rye berries.

### *Be skeptical of these tricky and easy-to-misinterpret words*

When you see the following words, you must investigate further, because some parts of the grain may possibly be missing: Wheat, wheat flour, semolina, durum wheat, organic flour, stone-ground, and multigrain. When in doubt, don't trust manufacturers of processed foods, because they may honestly be allowed to label the products as "wheat bread with whole grain" even if there is only a tiny amount of whole grain. Look for the ingredient's place on the list. If it's not in first place, it's unlikely to be whole grain.

### *More misleading words*

When you see these words, they do not describe whole grains: Enriched flour, degerminated corn meal, pearled or polished, and bran. Also, do not trust labels that say the food is high fiber when figuring out this whole grain business, because fiber (such as cellulose, which is a by-product of various wood industries and is useful for making things like cereal boxes) is a breeze to add to grains that have little nutritional value . . . and often is!

Don't make me name names here. If there is a cute television commercial telling you how the wife tricks the husband into eating delicious high-fiber food, because she is smart and he is a nitwit, it is unlikely to be from whole grains. Get your fiber from the source, not from additions.

*Specific common tricks currently being used*

Bread manufacturers love to call their product multi-grain when it is often white bread with a miniscule couple of whole grains thrown in. (And it's perfectly legal.) Wheat bread *is not* whole wheat bread, but rather white bread with some brown coloring added to make you think you're eating something healthy.

Pasta makers love this tricky wording, too, so double-check that your rice pasta is from brown rice, and your wheat pasta is whole wheat. Industry insiders know that the words wheat flour, enriched wheat flour, unbleached wheat flour, all-purpose flour, and enriched flour are all translated to mean white flour. Avoid if possible.

## THE BOTTOM LINE

Eat four to six servings of whole grain foods each day, and watch for labeling tricks meant to throw you off the trail of truly nutritious foods. Whole grains and complex carbohydrates are not the enemy. Quite the contrary, they are an important source of many of the nutrients required to keep our bodies in amazing working order.

There is a huge variety of whole grains available besides whole wheat. Try new grains such as those listed in the recipes section of this book. I've also included a handy chart from the Whole Grains Council that will tell you how to cook just about any grain, from amaranth to wild rice.

# 23. EAT FRESHLY-GROUND FLAXSEED DAILY

Flaxseed is a rich source of vitamins, minerals, and fiber. But wait, there's more! As if that isn't enough nutritional awesomeness for us, it is also the single richest source of plant phytoestrogens, weak hormones that plug up the receptors on cancer cells where estrogen wants to attach to feed your breast cancer.

This makes flaxseed one of the food items that we really ought to eat just about every day. It contains exceptionally high concentrations of lignans and is a rich source of a-linolenic acid, a polyunsaturated (omega-3 or "good") fatty acid.

Lignans are so similar to the female hormone estrogen that they compete with estrogen for a part in certain biologic actions. Consequently, natural estrogens seem to become less powerful, reducing unpleasant menopausal symptoms in many women, as lignans have been found to have anti-estrogenic effects.

Lilian Thompson and Jianmen Chen's names appear on much of the literature I reviewed in regard to flaxseed and breast cancer. Thompson and Chen, at the University of Toronto, have been studying the effects of flaxseed on the carcinogenesis of breast cancer for over a decade.

Their research team concluded in a review article in *Clinical Cancer Research* that there is strong evidence that flaxseed inhibits the growth of estrogen receptor positive breast cancer at both high and low estrogen levels (translating to pre- and postmenopausal estrogen levels, respectively).

The team found that flaxseed enhanced the effect of Tamoxifen against the growth of estrogen receptor positive human breast cancer in mice. Tamoxifen and flaxseed together reduced tumor growth by the dual actions of decreasing malignant cell growth and increasing cell death.

Eat fresh-ground flaxseed meal each day! We don't have the ability to metabolize whole flaxseed, so if they are consumed whole, they zip right on through our systems with little or no estrogenic effect. Buy it in the whole form. It comes in golden and black varieties; golden is typically more expensive but doesn't do anything different than the black.

Grind up a day's worth in the morning and try to use it as soon as you can as it tends to get rancid very quickly, even in the refrigerator. If rancid, it has a strong off-smell that reminds me of boiled linseed oil. Once ground, I begin the day by throwing it in or on whatever I'm eating for breakfast, whether a smoothie, or a tofu scramble, or hot cereal, and I put the remainder in a little container that I carry with me so that I can sprinkle it on my food throughout the rest of the day.

You will find that flaxseed meal makes for a reasonable egg replacement in recipes for baked goods. These are often referred to as "flax eggs" and they will not only bind your baked goods together in an admirable way, but will also amp up the nutritional value of whatever you put it in. You can find a recipe for flax eggs at the back of the book.

Start slow if you aren't used to eating a great deal of fiber yet, and remember to drink lots of water when you do. Otherwise, you may have to deal with an unpleasant case of constipation, so drink up and bulk up!

### THE BOTTOM LINE

Eat two to three tablespoons of fresh-ground flaxseed each day, but remember to start slow if this is a new part of your diet.

One final note: Don't take medication or supplements of any kind within an hour (before or after) of eating flaxseed, as it has been found to have the effect of washing meds through your system too quickly for them to be properly absorbed.

# 24. KICK SUGAR TO THE CURB

Our bodies have evolved over eons to have a natural craving for the taste of sweet, succulent fruits. We are drawn to them for a very good reason: They are packed to near-bursting with health-bestowing nutrients and supply powerful anti-aging, antioxidant, and anti-cancer properties.

Unfortunately, with the technology to extract the sweet sugar from the fruit (and sometimes, veggies, like sugar beets), came the ability to easily satisfy this healthy craving with unhealthy substitutes.

Candy, pastries, ice cream, and other sweets that are devoid of nutrition, fiber, or substance have come to fill our diets. According to the USDA, the average American in 1822 consumed 6.2 pounds of sugar a year. With that number now estimated at just over 75 pounds, it's no wonder we are now faced with an epidemic of obesity, diabetes, and lifestyle-related diseases, including breast cancer.

*Does sugar feed cancer?*

One of the first topics I found myself researching after diagnosis was whether sugar feeds cancer, as has been hypothesized for many years. I found the answer to be that, no, sugar does not feed cancer—at least not directly, it doesn't. But it most certainly *does* feed metabolic syndromes, including obesity and subsequent states of inflammation, which are flashing neon welcome signs to cancer cells.

All sugars, including honey, raw sugar, brown sugar, the Frankenfood high fructose corn syrup, and even molasses, as well as drinks that are primary providers of sugar, including both soft drinks and mass-produced fruit juices, provide substantial calories to your body with zero nutritional benefit.

Processed sugar serves no nutritional purpose: It's pure entertainment. And I don't know about you, but when I eat a gigantic Milky Way, my next nutritional move is unlikely to be a steaming plate of fresh kale.

## The science

In 2009, a large study confirmed that there is a link between the quantity of high-sugar, highly processed food and an increased risk of breast cancer. The risk increased point for point with a diet higher in simple carbohydrates, which we know leads to the release of hormones, such as insulin-like growth factors and insulin, into the bloodstream, and come from sugar, white flour, pastries, white rice, and sweets.

In another study, women with breast cancer who had the highest levels of insulin were twice as likely to relapse and three times more likely to develop metastases than those whose diets contained less sugar, and, therefore, had lower insulin levels in their blood.

And finally, in a massive 2009 study, researchers at the Albert Einstein College of Medicine observed over 90,000 women, concluding that the link between obesity and breast cancer is likely due to higher levels of insulin and estrogen in women with BMIs over 30.

## Just say no to artificial sweeteners

Zero or low calorie sodas and other processed food items that are sweetened with aspartame have been proven to contribute to weight gain, working in opposition to all of the good nutritional and exercise choices you are making by triggering sugar cravings. It also stimulates hunger in general.

## A few thoughts on agave

I know there are many who love agave nectar and think that they are doing a good thing by using it as a sweetener. The marketers of this stuff would have you believe that you are buying a raw and healthy sweetening product. However, most agave nectar is produced in a super-high-heat process that enlists the help of nasty caustic acids, clarifiers, and filtration chemicals.

Use with caution, and know your source: None of the agave found in your grocery store, and few found on the shelves of health food stores, are produced via the old artisanal process that does not rely on toxic chemistry.

## THE BOTTOM LINE

Generally speaking, use added sweeteners in moderation, and when you do need to sweeten, avoid highly chemically-processed products, agave nectar, high fructose corn syrup, and white sugar. Look to naturally made products from reliable sources such as coconut sugar and other less refined sweeteners, and sweeten lightly. These are much less likely to contribute to an inflammatory state and are surely a better fit with the health and nutritional goals you have set for yourself.

# 25. STRIVE TO ELIMINATE ANIMAL PROTEIN

One of my nutrition superheroes, T. Colin Campbell, believes in one simple truth. He believes if you want to change your health, you really need to change just one big thing: Your diet. He and colleagues at Cornell University have researched the connections between animal fat and a litany of health issues, reaching conclusions that have turned what we thought we knew about nutrition completely on its head.

Over and over, they found that higher consumption of meat, milk (including products made from it), and eggs is associated with a higher risk of all kinds of cancers, including breast cancer. In animal studies, Campbell and colleagues found that dietary protein "proved to be so powerful in its effect that we could turn on and turn off cancer growth simply by changing the level of protein consumed."

Casein, in particular, was found to support every single stage of cancer progression. Casein makes up 87% of cows' milk protein and is used in other dairy products, such as cheese and yogurt. It also shows up as a hidden ingredient in a wide variety of processed foods.

On the other side of this body of work lies another truth that has been found just as many times: Plant protein, found in nuts, seeds, beans, legumes, veggies, and yes, even in fruit, does not promote cancer growth of any kind, even at high levels of consumption.

*"But where do you get your protein?"*

I wish someone would give me a big ol' hug every time I've heard the question, "But where do you get your protein if you don't eat meat or dairy?" because I'd be the happiest woman that ever lived. (Or maybe it's possible I just like hugs. Either way.) I always answer these generally-but-not always-

107

well-meaning people with two questions: "How many grams of protein do *you* eat every day?" and "How many grams of protein does the USDA recommend?" (No one I have ever asked those two questions has had answers, by the way. I was thinkin' that someone so clearly worried about my nutrition would know these things. Just an observation.)

You will get a sufficient amount of protein on a whole foods, plant-based diet. The USDA calculates the Recommended Daily Allowance (RDA) of protein at .8 grams per kilogram of body weight. A woman weighing 68.2 kilograms (or 150 pounds, as we like to say here in the US) requires about 54.56 grams of protein a day to keep the machinery running properly, which is ridiculously easy to get.

Listen up, ladies, there is no protein deficiency happening anywhere near the bountiful plates of delicious food that can soon be providing your delightful daily nourishment. While it may seem, to many, that animal flesh, milk, eggs, and other dairy products deliver good-quality protein, this protein is delivered at a huge nutritional and medical cost: Saturated fat.

Our goal as in the saturated fat department is zero, and we want to increase fiber intake. Animal flesh, milk, and dairy are loaded with saturated fat and contribute zero fiber. That's zero. These foods simply don't meet our nutritional requirements in a pragmatic analysis of the facts. (Pasture-fed meat is more nutritionally sound, however, it still contains no fiber.)

The life-sustaining protein we require is found in all foods, in varying amounts, and this includes vegetables! We are fed this line of pure baloney that protein only comes from animal products, or that we have to combine foods to make them complete, which just does not stand up to scientific scrutiny.

*Protein combining debunked*

In the relatively ancient days of nutritional science, it was thought that people eating plant-based diets needed to perform confusing, elaborate, and magical "combining" exercises in order to produce "quality protein." This has been soundly and completely dismantled, debunked, and disproved.

If you eat a wide variety of fruits, vegetables, nuts, seeds, grains, and legumes, you will have ample building blocks of protein, and at the same time, you will increase the statistical odds that you will never have to answer that phone call from the doctor's office ever, ever, ever, again. And that, my dears, is a good thing.

*So where DO we get our plant-based protein?*

A wide variety of delicious plant-based whole foods will provide all of the protein required by a human adult. To follow are some of the major ways a plant-based diet provides more than adequate protein.

I'd like to stress that each of the following refers to a 100 gram portion, which is roughly an overflowing half-cup size, or up to 2/3 of a cup, depending on the density of the item. I really wanted this to be an apples-to-apples comparison, even though some of the foods on the list would not be consumed in a portion of that size, such as spirulina and flaxseeds.

*Gram-to-gram comparisons of plant-based protein sources*

*Spirulina* contains 57 grams of protein. It is a blue-green algae and a highly bioavailable and complete plant protein, containing all essential amino acids. You are unlikely to eat 100 grams of spirulina as it is high in sodium, because it's from the ocean. (So please don't.) It is generally added in very small quantities to smoothies and other foods for a nice protein bump: One tablespoon tossed into a smoothie would contribute 4 grams of protein.

*Peanuts, almonds, other nuts and seeds, and nut butters* generally have between 18 and 24 grams of protein. That's between five and seven grams of protein per ounce, which is roughly 28 peanuts, 16 to 18 cashews, or 24 almonds.

*Tempeh (tem-pay)* contains 18 grams of protein. I love tempeh, but I have to admit that for many years, I ate it only grudgingly, because I didn't know how to cook it properly. Check out the recipe section of this book for more information on cooking tempeh.

Tempeh is a fermented soybean-based food, a protein-packed alternative to its non-fermented cousin, tofu. It's great on a sandwich and doubles as a tasty alternative to meatballs in pasta, or over brown rice and vegetables. I often slice one chunk of tempeh into four sandwich-size portions and bake it in barbeque sauce. There are tons of recipes out there for tempeh bacon as well, including one in the last chapter of this book.

*Whole soybeans*, although high in fat, are one of the richest sources of protein on the planet, just below tempeh at 17 grams. Toss a handful on a large salad, and you have a satisfying and nutritious meal. *Edamame (edda-mah-may)* are green soybeans, often still in the pod, which are steamed and salted and eaten as a snack. They provide 11 grams of protein.

*Whole oats* are also high on the plant-based protein list at 17 grams.

*Seitan (say-tan)* has 16 grams of protein. It's more delicious, foolproof, and cost-effective (although a little bit of a time-consuming task) to make it yourself. Seitan is an excellent substitute for a newbie plant-based eater who is jonesing for beef, as it has roughly the same texture and tooth, as well as a similar protein count, ounce for ounce.

This is not a good protein for those with gluten sensitivities as the primary ingredient in seitan is vital wheat gluten. You will find a basic recipe by Chef Skye Michael in the recipe section of *Ultimate Survivorship*.

*Flaxseed, hemp seed, and chia seed* have 16 grams of protein, although that would be a ridiculously large serving. They have excellent ratios of omega-6 and omega-3 EFAs, making them highly bioavailable. These seeds are especially easy to add to hot breakfast cereals and baked goods. Chia seeds do not need to be ground up (but you can, and I have) and have some interesting gelling properties, making them a common addition to puddings or smoothies.

*Tofu (toe-foo)* contains 10 grams of protein. I serve it diced and broiled or toss it into soup for a protein boost. I have a mock egg salad recipe that my friends and family swear is the real thing, and it's made with tofu. It can be sliced, marinated, and made into sandwiches: It's versatile and delicious.

Tofu is known for its mild and unobtrusive flavor, which makes it a good candidate for mixing and matching with any other foods. If you freeze it and then thaw it, tofu will take on a chewy, meaty texture that makes a perfect substitute for ground beef.

*Lentils* are a real protein powerhouse at nine grams. They are super-delicious, super-nutritious, and super-easy to prepare. Green lentils, sometimes referred to as French lentils, are very firm and hold up well in soups, stews, and salads.

Other lentils, usually shades of brown or orange, will cook down to more of a mushy consistency, but that's a good thing as they thicken up soup nicely and make great veggie burgers for the same reason.

*Beans and split peas* have between eight and nine grams of protein and are fiber champs to boot. There are a huge variety of beans available including soybeans, cannellini, small white, black, kidney, mung, pinto, black-eyed peas, adzuki, garbanzos, and fava, to name just a few.

I usually start with dry beans and cook them in economical big batches in a pressure cooker (because they are a breeze to freeze), but always keep cans of them at work and at home for quick-fast meal prep. They are perfect on burritos, in chili and soups, on greens, or over quinoa or brown rice.

Beans, beans, the musical fruit, I do adore them and they are on my plate every day. Pre-soaking dry beans and tossing the soak-water will help with the music factor quite a bit. Because they are such a fiber powerhouse, if you aren't used to eating beans, start slow, and let your system adjust.

*Quinoa (keen-wah)* contains four grams of protein, which is the same amount as an equal portion of chicken breast. Quinoa is a small grain-like seed with a super-high protein profile that contains all of the amino acids, making it a perfect protein. It is one of the fastest grains to get to the table at around 15 minutes.

Quinoa is a one-to-one substitute for rice or pasta, served alone or with vegetables and greens. It squishes up and can hold together really well and thus makes excellent veggie burgers; it works well in pilafs, or with cinnamon, maple syrup, and nut milk as a hot cereal. It has a very mild, nutty flavor and a little bit of a satisfying crunch no matter how long it's cooked.

Quinoa is truly one of my go-to staple foods. When using, rinse well, and then rinse again, as it is covered in a bitter substance that keeps birds from eating it. Some brands advertise that they are "pre-washed."

*Vegetables and dried fruit* Even veggies have protein, as I mentioned, and while not as much as other sources, you simply cannot deny the additional protein they bring to the table. From sweet green peas at five grams of protein to avocado, broccoli, Brussels sprouts, spinach, cauliflower, watercress, potato with the skin on, asparagus, and dried fruit, at between two and three grams, all will add unexpected protein.

This includes all types of sprouts, including alfalfa, mung bean, and radishes. I also noted while doing this research that dried fruits are a source of protein that their fresh counterparts are not, for some reason.

*Mushrooms* are another adequate source of protein. Portabella mushrooms and good ol' white button mushrooms each provide four grams, while shiitake mushrooms provide two grams.

*Whole grains* Even these, sitting at the bottom of the plant-based protein list, will add to the variety being eaten on this particular diet. Whole wheat and rye breads come in at 13 and eight grams (four and three per slice, respectively) and whole wheat spaghetti at five, with most other grains hovering around three grams of protein per serving.

## THE BOTTOM LINE

A high-quality, high-quantity whole foods, plant-based diet will provide more than adequate protein for one human adult female who wishes to nourish herself like the queen that she really is. Meat and dairy in general, and casein in particular, have been shown to be powerful cancer promoters. Strive to eliminate all sources of animal protein from your diet.

# 26. LEARN TO COOK WITH LITTLE OR NO ADDED FAT

Our bodies are complicated and intricate systems within systems within systems, working together, reacting to minute biological changes, always seeking stasis, and relying on resources that are often shared. I now know this is a delicate, intricate mechanism such that when one part is out of whack, another system, sometimes one that you wouldn't think is related, can fly out of whack, too.

We are made up of these amazing webs of actions and reactions, and that's one of the biggest Big Ideas I've grappled with and come to understand recently. We can't just toss down a pill to fix what's broken. We can't just do one thing. We gotta fix the entire system, because there is no such thing as a system that acts on its own. That is such a simple and elegant thing, I could almost cry sometimes. I really mean that.

Although time-consuming, the act of gathering up all of the information out there on the topic of breast cancer has not been the trickiest part of this whole "never again!" business I'm in. Putting it all together into a cohesive plan, now there's the real trick.

This task has been daunting at times, and at others, confusing, and sometimes there is what appears to be conflicting information floating around. But if you pay attention, and listen to the experts, a pattern emerges, and everything becomes somewhat simpler.

The topic of dietary fat is just such a confusing topic, and it is teeming with what appears to be conflicting advice. Early on, I decided that the expert I would rely on for any particular area of research would be the one with the most depth of experience. No matter the study, no matter the science, the reality remains that disentangling truth from a scientific study can sometimes be an art form unto itself. For this I rely on the experts.

113

There have been two large studies that looked at dietary fat and breast cancer in great depth. Participants in the Women's Intervention Nutrition Study (WINS), whose diets consisted of 20% fat (considered low-fat), were found to have a 24% reduction of metastasis. Much discussion ensued after the study, in which some said the reduction came from the average six pound weight loss the women also reported. There may be infighting in the scientific community, but to this, I say: Whatever the reason is, whether it's the weight or the fat, I'm just fine with the outcome.

The other, the Women's Healthy Eating and Living (WHEL) study, was the second largest observational analysis of diet and breast cancer. In this, the women reported fat calories were 26.9% of their diets (larger than the first study, but still significantly lower than most American diets). Breast cancer prognosis again improved.

There has also been debate and discussion surrounding this study in the scientific community, but, honestly, I can't imagine how difficult it would be to decide which parts of women's diets were the causative factor and which were not. Teasing those things out from what is referred to as an observational study (asking women to report on their behavior) is a daunting task, I would think. That's just another reason to look at these studies for clues and directions that make common sense.

There is a professional lifetime body of work to refer to in the area of dietary fat and breast cancer, and the expert whose advice I follow in this area of nutrition is Dr. Mary Flynn. Her research supports the use of what could be called a modified Mediterranean diet that includes small amounts of omega-3 olive oil, not only for maximum nutrition, but for weight loss effectiveness, as well.

Her 2010 findings, reported in the *Journal of Women's Health*, were that an olive oil-enriched diet brought about greater weight loss than a low-fat diet in an eight week comparison. Moreover, the study participants overwhelmingly chose the olive oil diet for six months of follow-up. In my opinion, it is vitally important that we feel satisfied by the food we eat in order to carry any changes forward long-term.

An Israeli study published in the *New England Journal of Medicine* backed up the team's findings. Over a period of two years, women lost more weight and had measurable changes for the better in biomarkers for breast cancer, including blood lipids, blood sugar, and insulin, on a plant-based olive oil diet.

And finally, a significant study, published in 2006 in the *New England Journal of Medicine* confirmed what cardiovascular researchers have been telling us for years: Trans-fats are bad for us! These are the processed oils (hydrogenated and partially hydrogenated) found in many industrially-concocted foods.

*Vegetables, including tomatoes, and olive oil*

The lycopene in tomatoes is made more available with the addition of a little bit of olive oil, which is an essential component of our health plan on other levels as well. A salad dressing made with a small amount of extra virgin olive oil, or a little bit of olive oil drizzled on roasted vegetables, will greatly increase the nutritional value. (Adding avocado, nuts, and seeds to your salad will accomplish the same thing.)

Purdue researcher Mario Ferruzzi found that while you may have a reduction in calories when using a fat-free salad dressing, you are losing some of the benefits of the veggies at the same time. Ferruzzi's team of researchers fed the study participants salads with either saturated, monounsaturated, or polyunsaturated fat-based dressings.

They were then tested for fat-soluble nutrients found in the veggies they had eaten. It was determined that monounsaturated was the best at releasing the greatest amount of carotenoids with the least amount of fat. Olive oil is the most common type of this fat.

*Use organic, cold-pressed, extra-virgin olive oil*

It is worth the little extra money you have to dole out to get the best quality olive oil you can afford, especially given the small amount of oil you will be using. Most of the inexpensive oils on the typical grocery shelf are processed at high temperatures and using toxic chemicals to extract the oils from the source, whether soybean, canola, olive, or others.

Only when you purchase cold-pressed and certified organic can you be assured that the extra-virgin olive oil in your pantry is the healthiest available. Buy it in small bottles and keep it in the refrigerator.

## THE BOTTOM LINE

It will serve us well to avoid the slathering on and misuse of added fats and to follow a low-fat diet. Our goal is 10-25% of our food in healthy fats, with zero saturated (animal) fats. Include very small amounts (no more than one to two tablespoons per day) of cold-pressed organic extra virgin olive oil in your salad dressings and when cooking vegetables, to increase the bioavailability of important phytochemicals, feel fuller, and enjoy increased long-term dietary success.

# 27. EAT A WIDE VARIETY OF
# VEGGIES, FRUITS, AND OTHER PLANTS

Here we are, finally and at long-last, at the place where I get to talk about the lip-smacking, rainbow-colored, crunchy-crispy, sweet-tart, luscious heart and belly-rubbing soul of our anti-breast cancer sustenance—veggies, fruits, and other plants!

Momma always said to "eat your veggies, they're good for you!" and although she might not have known how or exactly why, Momma was absolutely right, unless she thought that gloppy mess known as green bean casserole was a vegetable. No judgment here, just information. (Awright, awright, I'm judging this processed-salty-glopfest more than just a little. Yuck!)

I don't know about yours, but my Momma's admonition was a combination of guesswork and common sense. Today, that is also backed up by nutritional and biochemical science. This is no time for half-baked efforts. This is about long-term survival, and science gives us very specific instructions as to which specific foods will have the greatest effect on our very specific cancer. This isn't simply an anti-cancer plan, no, ma'am, it is an anti-breast cancer plan.

A team of researchers conducted an analysis of eight different studies, accounting for over 80% of the findings in regard to carotenoids (found in fruits and veggies) and their effect on breast cancer cells. In more than 3,000 of the 3,055 cases studied, the team found a statistically significant correlation between higher levels of circulating carotenoids and a decreased risk of breast cancer.

Reported in the *Journal of the National Cancer Institute* in December of 2012, the team concluded that women with higher levels of alpha-carotene, beta-carotene, lutein+zeaxanthin, lycopene, and total carotenoids may be at reduced risk of breast cancer.

A similar study, conducted in Germany and reported in the *British Journal of Cancer* in November 2012, studied the dietary patterns of 2,500 breast cancer survivors. A healthy dietary pattern planned around a high intake of veggies and fruits was associated with reduced overall mortality and lower recurrence of the cancer.

## *Phytochemical heroes*

The heroes in all of these studies are phytochemicals, a term that refers to the variously chemically-active compounds found, naturally-occurring, in plants, including fruits, veggies, beans, legumes, grains, and other edible plant material.

There is some evidence that certain phytochemicals are responsible for preventing the formation of carcinogens in our bodies, for blocking the action of carcinogens that have already been formed, for blocking the actions of carcinogens on their targets in our bodies, and for suppressing cancer development once it has begun. Wow. Seriously.

## *Some important phytochemicals*

Flavonoids are any of a group of phytochemicals containing compounds that smell good to people and animals (which attracts us to them) and is widely distributed in plants, often as a pigment. They are found in a wide variety of grains, vegetables, and fruits, especially in those with colorful skins.

We know that oxidative damage plays a significant role in the development of cancer. The task of flavonoids is to counteract this damage, and, as a result, are antioxidant by nature. In addition, flavonoids have anti-inflammatory characteristics that result from their ability to inhibit the effects of pro-inflammatory compounds in our cells.

Flavonoids of special interest to breast cancer survivors are quercetin, apigenin, epigallocatechin (also known as ECGC), the group anthocyanins and anthocyanidins, and isoflavones. (There won't be a test. Please, just let this information kind of wash over you in a general way.)

Quercetin, found in apples, red and yellow onions, tea, wine, cranberries, buckwheat, and beans, has been found to have anti-breast cancer properties. In vitro studies have shown that they not only slow tumor cell growth, but also work to speed tumor cell death.

Apigenin, found in chamomile, celery, and parsley, appears to block the formation of new blood vessels in breast cancer tumors, which essentially cuts off the food supply, slowing down or even halting their development.

ECGC, found in green tea, has powerful antioxidant effects. The team performing a meta-analysis published in the journal *Carcinogenesis* in 2006 concluded that green tea consumption has a statistically significant effect on breast cancer. You will get more details about the amazing healing properties of green tea in a few more chapters, to be sure.

Anthocyanins and anthocyanidins, the most abundant of the flavonoids, are found in fruits noted for their intensely-colored red, purple, or blue skins, including bilberries, raspberries, strawberries, blueberries, cherries, cranberries, blackberries, peaches, plums, and eggplants. They have been shown to exhibit anti-cancer activity against multiple types of cancer cells.

Ellagic acid, belonging to another classification called phenolic acids, is found in walnuts, strawberries, cranberries, blackberries, guava, pomegranates, and grapes. It has been found to have a strong antioxidant effect and has been seen to slow the growth of some tumors in preliminary studies. It has been shown to inhibit the binding of carcinogens to DNA.

Stilbenoids are primarily found in deep blue and purple fruits. The most highly studied stilbenoid is resveratrol, which is found in grape skins and seeds, wine, nuts, peanuts, Japanese knotweed root, and blueberries. Resveratrol has antioxidant and anti-inflammatory properties, and may induce tumor cell death as well as playing a part in cell cycle and estrogen receptor function in breast cancer lines.

I almost hate to talk about resveratrol here because it is such a hyped-up supplement, and not only should you run out and start buying so-called "miracle supplements" such as this (or others) that will supposedly cure everything that ails you, but that is the direct opposite of what science tells us to do. Do not start taking this, or anything else, as a supplement. This just isn't a scientifically proven strategy. Instead, eat deep-colored grapes and occasionally drink a small glass of dark red wine.

Carotenoids are a huge group of phytochemicals with tremendous power against breast cancer. They are known, for the most part, by their orange and yellow pigments. In the carotene branch of carotenoids are alpha-carotene, found in carrots, pumpkins, maize, tangerines, and oranges, and beta-carotene, found in dark, leafy greens, and in red, orange, and yellow fruits and vegetables.

There is important research showing that carotenoids must come from the whole-food source. Taking them as supplements has been shown to have a negative effect on human health!

Lycopene is found in tomatoes, grapefruit, watermelon, guava, apricots, carrots, Vietnamese gac fruit, and autumn olive. While its role in breast cancer prevention is not clear, there is a known correlation to prevention of other types of cancers. It also aids in the synthesis of carotene.

Zeaxanthin is found in the yellow pigments, the xanthophylls, found in spinach, kale, turnip greens, maize, red pepper, pumpkin, wolfberry, and oranges, and lutein, found in spinach, turnip greens, romaine lettuce, red pepper, pumpkin, mango, papaya, oranges, kiwi, peaches, squash, legumes, brassicates (that's the broccoli gang), prunes, sweet potatoes, honeydew melon, rhubarb, plum, avocado, pear, and cilantro.

## *Isoflavones*

Isoflavones (*aka* phytoestrogens) are found in soy, alfalfa sprouts, red clover, chickpeas, peanuts, and other legumes. They work by binding to the estrogen receptor of tumor cells, which means that they essentially plug up holes that our own estrogen would normally be attracted to and that feed estrogen receptor positive cancer. They also have attributes not related to hormones, in that they encourage tumor cell death and inhibit tumor growth.

## *Turmeric and black pepper*

The compound curcumin is found in turmeric, which is the primary ingredient in the bright orange-gold Indian spice mixture curry. In 2005, researchers found that dietary curcumin significantly decreased the incidence of breast cancer metastasis to the lung and concluded that, as a pharmacologically safe compound, it has therapeutic potential in preventing breast cancer metastasis.

Dr. Madhuri Kakarala has completed research into the amazing and almost outlandish synergistic effect of curcumin together with piperine, found in fresh-cracked pepper. You'll hear more about her research in the chapter on spices.

## *Lignans*

Lignans are an important addition to anti-breast cancer diets. Another phytoestrogen, it is found in seeds (especially flaxseed, but also in chia, sesame, pumpkin, sunflower, and poppy), whole grains (especially rye, oats, and barley), bran (wheat, oat, and rye), fruits (particularly berries), and vegetables.

Case-controlled studies frequently show an association between regular dietary lignan consumption and reduction in breast cancer. It should be noted that the lignans present in flaxseed are not found in flaxseed oil (nor is there fiber in the oil).

## *Lipids*

Lipids are the fats and oils found in plants. Phytosterols are one category of lipids, absorbed in small amounts that nonetheless play a significant role in preventing breast cancer, and found in almonds, cashews, peanuts, seeds, whole wheat, maize, soybeans, and vegetable oils.

Current research suggests that an increased consumption of foods containing phytosterols is associated with reduced breast cancer risk. They enable more robust antitumor responses by our bodies, including the boosting of immune recognition of cancer cells, by influencing hormone-dependent tumor growth, and by altering the manufacture of female hormones by our bodies.

They have also been seen to have a direct effect on cancerous tumor growth, including the slowing of cell cycle progression, encouraging cell suicide, and the inhibition of metastasis.

## *. . . and more phytochemicals*

Organosulfides are some of our best defenses against all types of cancer, and not just against breast cancer. Of particular interest to us are isothiocyanates (ITCs), allium compounds, and sulfides.

The ITCs include sulforaphane, found in all brassicates, especially broccoli and broccoli sprouts, and have been shown to inhibit breast cancer circulating tumor cells. It is important that these particular substances are broken down by chopping, chewing, or blending, because this initiates chemical reactions that are protective against all types of cancers.

Eating the brassicates on a regular basis helps our bodies reduce the cancer-promoting potency of estrogen and other hormones and also helps with hormone excretion. Chinese women who ate one serving each day of cruciferous veggies reduced their breast cancer risk by over 50%. One of our best sources of sulforaphane is broccoli sprouts, with 100 times the concentration as it is in broccoli.

The brassicate family includes arugula, bok choy, broccoli, broccoli rabe, broccolini, Brussels sprouts, cabbage, cauliflower, collards, horseradish, kale, kohlrabi, mustard greens, radishes, rutabaga, turnips, turnip greens, and watercress.

ITCs detoxify and remove carcinogens, kill cancer cells, and prevent tumor growth by preventing new blood supply formation. They have more than just general anti-cancer properties. They are especially protective against hormone-related cancers like breast cancer.

The allium compounds are found in garlic, onions, leeks, chives, and shallots, and show promise as an addition to your breast cancer-fighting menu. The chemopreventive activity of garlic has been shown to be first class for all cancers, which has been attributed to the organosulfides present.

Diallyl disulfide (DADS) is an oil-soluble compound found in garlic, onions, leeks, chives, and shallots, which has been found to suppress breast cancer.

Indoles and glucosinolates/sulfur compounds are one last group of anti-breast cancer phytochemicals that are truly begging to be a part of your prevention plan. Especially important are indole-3-carbinol (I3C) and indole [3,2-b] carbazole (ICZ), which are the primary bioactive food components in cruciferous vegetables, including broccoli and cabbage.

Numerous studies have shown that I3C and ICZ have anti-breast cancer cellular effects. They inhibit tumor cell movement, have antiproliferative effects, and also have anti-estrogenic properties.

*New math: 4 X 1 = 20*

In another scientific paper on the topic, researcher Rui Hai Liu reported that the synergistic effects of phytochemicals in fruits and vegetables are responsible for their potent antioxidant and anti-cancer properties, and that the benefit of a diet rich in whole fruits and vegetables is attributed to the complex interactions of the phytochemicals present.

For example, the bioavailability of non-heme iron, found in spinach, is enhanced with the addition of ascorbic acid, or vitamin C.

Researchers at Cornell University found that a 1.75 ounce serving of apples, blueberries, grapes, and oranges had about five times the antioxidant power of each fruit on its own. Micronutrient synergy is a fascinating new area of scientific research, and I can't wait to hear about new synergies that will be found in the next few years.

## THE BOTTOM LINE

Eat seven to nine servings a day of nutrient-rich vegetables and fruits. It is important to focus on those vegetables that have been shown to specifically work for us as breast cancer survivors.

Garlic, scallions, and leeks are three of the top-rated vegetables for all cancers, including ours, for the allium compounds and DADS.

Make sure at least one or two of your veggie servings each day is from the cruciferous group, including arugula, bok choy, broccoli, broccoli rabe, broccolini, Brussels sprouts, cabbage, cauliflower, collards, horseradish, kale. kohlrabi, mustard greens, radishes, rutabaga, turnips, turnip greens,

122

and watercress, for sulforaphane, indoles, and glucosinolates/sulfur compounds.

Other fruits and veggies to eat include apples, red and yellow onions, and cranberries (for quercetin), celery and parsley (for apigenin), bilberries, raspberries, strawberries, blueberries, cherries, cranberries, blackberries, peaches, plums, and eggplants (for anthocyanins and anthocyanidins), strawberries, cranberries, blackberries, guava, pomegranates, and grapes (for ellagic acid), carrots, pumpkins, tangerines, and oranges (for carotene), dark, leafy greens, and red, orange, and yellow fruits and veggies (for beta-carotene), spinach, kale, turnip greens, red pepper, pumpkin, wolfberry, and oranges (for zeaxanthin), spinach, turnip greens, romaine lettuce, red pepper, pumpkin, mango, papaya, oranges, kiwi, peaches, squash, the brassicates (that's the broccoli-cauliflower-cabbage gang), prunes, sweet potatoes, honeydew melon, rhubarb, plum, avocado, pear, and cilantro (for lutein), alfalfa sprouts and red clover (for isoflavones).

The more you mix and match colors, the more your body will have to work with in the way of anti-cancer superfood building blocks. Eating more than one veggie or fruit at the same time seems to have an amazing synergistic effect as well, so make sure to mix it up!

,

# 28. EAT MUSHROOMS

Mushrooms have been honored for hundreds of years, not only for the flavor and texture they bring to our diets, but for their gentle yet powerful nutritional value. They have been widely appreciated, primarily in Eastern practice, for a number of biochemical properties: Mushrooms are antioxidant and antidiabetic; they fight cholesterol, are antimicrobial, and, of particular interest to breast cancer survivors, they not only support immune function but have both anti-cancer and antitumor properties. This is a true anti-breast cancer superfood.

There is a growing body of scientific evidence suggesting that eating common dietary mushrooms that are readily available in most grocery stores can reduce breast cancer risk and recurrence, including maitake, cremini, portobello, oyster, and yes, even the lowly white button mushroom. In a prominent study of Chinese women with breast cancer, daily consumption of 10 grams of fresh button mushrooms (that's roughly one) significantly decreased the risk of breast cancer in both pre- and postmenopausal women.

Mushrooms are believed to be protective against all types of cancers, but protect against breast cancer in particular because they inhibit an enzyme called aromatase, which produces estrogen. Many breast cancer survivors take medication that inhibits aromatase production, depending on their menopausal status. Two mushroom varieties that have been shown to have aromatase activity are white button and portobello.

Mushrooms of all varieties contain particular phytochemicals that perform anti-cancer cartwheels, including lectin, b-glucan, ergosterol, and arginine.

Lectin inhibits the growth of tumor cells, reduces the rate of proliferation of breast cancer cells, suppresses tumors by speeding along cell death cycles, and induces an immune response.

B-glucan directly inhibits tumor cell growth, represses cancer progression, hinders metastatic progress, lessens the expression of tumor markers, and increases natural killer (NK) cell activity. NK cells work just like it sounds they might—our very own ninja force, running around and disabling the bad guys.

B-glucan also enhances the immune system, reduces proliferation and viability of breast cancer cells, stimulates blood monocytes in patients with advanced breast cancer, inhibits the growth of tumor cells, affects the expression of several important genes in breast cancer cells, inhibits cell proliferation, and suppresses the metastatic behavior of breast cancer cells.

Ergosterol slows tumor growth by inhibiting its blood supply and exhibits a powerful anti-migratory effect on breast cancer cells.

Arginine inhibits tumor growth, reduces nitrogen losses, contributes to a positive nitrogen balance, has an anti-proliferation effect, and improves anti-cancer biological activity.

There is a huge variety of mushrooms available. Baby bellas (sometimes called brown or cremini mushrooms) look like common white button mushrooms but have a firmer texture and stronger yet still mild flavor. They can be used in any dish calling for mushrooms.

Chanterelles have a fruity aroma and delicate taste and can be orange, yellow, brown, black, or even white, with funnel-shaped caps that have wrinkles instead of gills.

Oyster mushrooms are more trumpet-shaped and can have light brown, gray, or reddish caps, with lighter stems and a peppery flavor that becomes milder when cooked. They are great in stir-fries, soups, and sauces.

Shiitakes have a chewy, meaty texture and smoky flavor with tan or dark brown caps. They have been fairly extensively studied as immune-boosters. The stems can be tough but are great in vegetable stocks or soups (just strain them out of the stock or fish them out of the soup before serving).

Portobellos have a great-big, beefy flavor and texture, and for that reason are often used as veggie burgers. They are excellent on the grill and on a bun with all the toppings. The stems can be a bit woody, but save them in the freezer for your stock pot, or chop them up small for soup.

And finally, white button are the most common mushrooms on the market. They have a more delicate taste and texture than portobello or cremini mushrooms. Don't let their lack of color fool you into thinking they aren't nutritious. They are!

*Turkey tail mushrooms*

A phase one clinical study reported in 2012 in the journal *ISRN Oncology* suggested that turkey tail mushrooms are a safe immunotherapy for breast cancer patients, noting that "relapse after primary breast cancer treatment may be related to defects in the innate and adaptive immune system," adding that turkey tail mushrooms could have significant applications for breast cancer survivors. These can be purchased dried and made into tea or used as an ingredient.

### Mushrooms and vitamin D

Mushrooms are also a source of vitamin D, which is frequently deficient in breast cancer patients. Researchers at Boston University School of Medicine found that exposing mushrooms (after they have been picked) to UV radiation creates an abundant source of vitamin D, comparable to that found in supplements. A few commercial growers are taking advantage of this new information, increasing the nutritional value of their product in just this manner.

If you want to do it yourself (like I do, because it's usually cheaper and almost always better) you can simply place your sliced mushrooms gill-side-up in direct sunlight for a half an hour prior to cooking them. For a more time-intensive project, you can also lay your sliced mushrooms in the sun for two full days, and then finish drying them in a food dehydrator. When you are ready to eat them, simply rehydrate. The vitamin D does not dissipate when stored in this way.

According to head researcher Michael Hollick and his co-authors, eating mushrooms prepared in this way can enhance your vitamin D status. "The observation that some mushrooms, when exposed to UVB light, also produce vitamin D3 and vitamin D4 can also provide the consumer with at least two additional vitamin Ds," according to Hollick.

### Mushrooms and green tea

We know that regular consumption of mushrooms is associated with a decreased risk of breast cancer. In one large Chinese study, women who ate the equivalent of about one cooked mushroom a day had a 64% decreased risk of breast cancer. Adding the synergistic power of green tea to the diet resulted in an 82% reduction in the same risk for menopausal women.

### THE BOTTOM LINE

Mushrooms have nutritional, antioxidant and immune-boosting characteristics. Include them in your meals often!

# 29. GET SPICY

Ah, spices, I love you so! I'd bust out singing a love song . . . but you are going to have to believe me when I say that everyone's much better off if that doesn't happen, so I'll say this instead: If good, wholesome food is the heart of the anti-breast cancer lifestyle, then spices are the passionate, pulsating soul. And I don't say that simply because of the flavors that good quality spices bring to the table.

As a result of burgeoning issues associated with chronic diseases that have ties to diet and lifestyle, researchers are constantly adding to a body of epidemiologic evidence that points not just to foods, but to culinary spices and herbs as important and inexpensive cancer mediators.

There is little real data about effective and safe dosages for the spices that are making their way into the headlines, with wild fluctuations in potencies from crop to crop and location to location, so I am not talking about actual supplementation with any of these spices. This discussion is about adding a wide variety of organic, non-irradiated herbs and spices to your food on a daily basis.

I do expect to start hearing about supplementation and dosing for at least a few of these spices in the years to come, but let's leave that to the scientific community to decide. Hang tight until the researchers figure that aspect out for us. Meanwhile, remember that little things add up and that oftentimes very small additions can become powerfully strong when the synergy of food micronutrients comes into play.

Spices come from the roots, flowers, fruits, seeds, or bark of a plant—as opposed to herbs, which come just from the leaves and are, generally speaking, less potent—and contain phytochemicals, the same types of compounds that we learned about when talking about fruits and vegetables, but for the most part, these compounds are intensified in spices. It's what gives them their flavor and makes them useful to us on so many different levels.

P.S. I'm not going to get all tied up in whether something is an herb or a spice, and I hope you'll go along with me on that.

There are five primary roles that spices play in our anti-cancer routines. They act as modifiers of the microbial environment (either stimulating the good microbes or inhibiting the bad ones), as antioxidants, as anti-inflammatory agents, and as cancer cell and tumor suppressors. There is scant research regarding the antimicrobial role and breast cancer (apparently there is a role for spices in this aspect for many gastric-type cancers, but that's a different discussion) so I'm just going to focus on the other four.

## Antioxidant

Humans require oxygen for most of the metabolic functions of these biologic super-systems we call home. In these systemic processes, the oxygen molecule that has been used gives off one (or more) electrons, which leaves them in a state of imbalance. These are the famous free radicals, whose time is spent running around looking in vain for their missing molecules.

If not ushered out of the body by antioxidants, they will grab whatever cellular tissue they can, wreaking havoc, disrupting normal, healthy cellular activities, leading to unhealthy tissues and to DNA damage, which not only compromises our immunity but can easily lead not only to cancer but to faster aging of all of our systems.

Think of this process as another type of oxidation that we are all very familiar with: Rust. You can see the visible damage done to metals by the oxidation process, and if you could see your cells, you would see oxidative stress there as well. It makes sense that if we can use tasty spices to flood our bodies with oxidant scavengers to clear the bad guys out, we really might want to give it a go.

## Anti-inflammatory

Since our friend Virchow first suggested a possible link between inflammation and cancer in 1863, it has been estimated that inflammation plays a role in about 15% of all cancers. As we know, inflammation in and of itself does not cause cancer, but it has been shown to create an environment in which cancer is able to thrive. Because there are so many side effects associated with aspirin and other anti-inflammatory drugs, it is reasonable that we have begun to turn to the common and safe compounds in spices for help.

*Halting carcinogen bioactivation*

Certain enzymes play a role in the activation of procarcinogens in our bodies that are not necessarily going to cause cancer, but are ripe and ready to be altered by some metabolic process to activate it. Some enzymes may hurt us by activating these procarcinogens and others help us by showing these nasty critters to the door. Many phytochemicals in spices have been shown to have an inhibitory effect on these metabolic processes that can ignite cancer cells.

*Anti-tumor*

Tumor growth can be activated by carcinogens in our environment, by inflammation, and by other metabolic processes. Certain pathways in particular play important roles in promoting breast cancer tumors, and once again, the phytochemicals in spices can inhibit and sometimes bring about changes in these pathways that regulate cell division, cell proliferation, and detoxification.

*Turmeric*

Turmeric sits right at the very top of my Anti-Breast Cancer Honor Roll of Spices. One study, published in the *Journal of Biological Chemistry*, reported that curcumin, the phytochemical in turmeric, may improve the effectiveness of some chemotherapy drugs. Another, in the journal *Clinical Cancer Research*, reported that curcumin suppressed a pathway that assists the growth of head and neck cancers. Numerous other studies have shown that curcumin is a powerful breast cancer preventive agent.

*Turmeric plus black pepper*

Even more recently, a team of researchers at the University of Michigan found that curcumin and piperine, the phytochemical found in freshly-cracked black pepper, separately and in combination inhibit breast cancer stem cell self-renewal through the inhibition of pathway signaling needed by the cancer cells. According to lead researcher Madhuri Kakarala, current therapies do not work against cancer stem cells, which is why cancer recurs and spreads.

She believes that eliminating these stem cells is an important key to preventing breast cancer metastasis. Curcumin and piperine both have substantial clinical research backing up their use as antioxidants, as anti-inflammatories, and as cancer preventatives, but this particular study was

131

groundbreaking in that it was the first to suggest that they could prevent cancer by targeting stem cells. (Stem cells are those unspecialized cells that can give rise to any type of cell, which is important because breast cancer stem cells feed tumor growth.) Kakarala found that the addition of pepper to the turmeric improved the bioavailability of the curcumin substantially.

What does this mean to us as breast cancer survivors? It means that someday there will be a safe dose of turmeric and black pepper for my two beautiful daughters (and yours), and very soon, I hope it means that it will be a potent and safe breast cancer preventative. It also means that I keep turmeric in a place of honor in my kitchen, sprinkling it on much of my food, and in as many recipes as I can reasonably manage, along with fresh ground cracked pepper.

### Freshly-ground, please!

Always use fresh-ground pepper when possible, as the volatile substances in this spice dissipate in about an hour once ground up and exposed to the air. (It tastes a thousand times better, too. That's a less-than-scientific fact, but a fact it is.) You can add a teensy bit of olive oil to your turmeric-black pepper combination to increase bioavailability even further.

### Ginger

The active phytochemical in ginger is gingerol, a relative of the substance capsaicin in peppers that gives this breast cancer inhibitor its characteristic zing. Many have used ginger through the ages for its anti-inflammatory and anti-nausea abilities, but it is (of course) the breast cancer prevention properties that are of primary interest to us.

A study published in the *Journal of Biomedicine and Biotechnology* in 2012 concluded that ginger could be a very promising candidate for the treatment of breast cancer carcinomas. The researchers discovered that ginger had the ability to have an impact on a "surprisingly wide variety of molecular mechanisms simultaneously," including assisting with cancer cell death, stimulating cell death, down-regulating cancer-related proteins, and encouraging increased expression of cancer inhibitors. This new information comes on the heels of many other studies that show ginger to be an effective breast-cancer inhibitor.

### The leafy herbs

There is a large group of herbs in the labiate family that are a welcome addition to our cancer-fighting cupboard, including rosemary, mint, thyme, marjoram, oregano, sage, and basil, among others. There are many studies concluding that these tasty herbs demonstrate high antioxidant activity.

## *Cloves*

Studies have shown that one of the phytochemicals in the spice clove, eugenol, has powerful antioxidant properties and, in one study, exhibited the strongest free radical scavenging activity among 26 spices tested.

## THE BOTTOM LINE

Herbs and spices all have phytochemical properties that result from the chemical properties of their differing flavor essences. Use them freely, mix and match, and experiment with new tastes. While turmeric and black pepper is the top-shelf spice combination that breast cancer survivors can look to regarding its healthful properties, use a generous hand with all herbs and spices, and as always, expect synergies to happen when you combine more than one.

# 30. EAT MODERATE AMOUNTS
# OF WHOLE ORGANIC SOY

One very tasty way to nourish yourself (in the healthy protein department) is the blank slate (in the taste department) soy. Soybeans are not only a rich source of protein, but they are abundantly blessed with isoflavones, a major group of phytoestrogens that have been shown to have protective benefits for breast cancer survivors when consumed in moderate amounts.

At one time, not that long ago, there was fairly substantial controversy in the scientific community regarding soy. As plant-food with mild "estrogen-like" effects, there was some concern that it would promote estrogen-fed breast cancer, and some caution was advised by the oncology community. Because the isoflavones in soy are phytoestrogens, the concern was that they would mimic estrogen in our systems, which, of course, would be a bad thing for those of us with estrogen receptor positive cancer.

Evidence began to mount that the opposite was true, and in December 2009, the *Journal of the American Medical Association* presented the findings of the Shanghai Breast Cancer Survival Study, a large Chinese cohort study of 5,042 breast cancer survivors. In that group, soy food consumption was significantly associated with a decreased risk of both death and recurrence of breast cancer.

*Eating soy is "statistically relevant" for decreased recurrence*

There issued additional concern in the scientific community that these results might not extrapolate to American women with their western diets, as we are not generally raised eating tofu and tempeh. More study was called for. These concerns were allayed with the release of the analysis of three large cohort studies, published in the May 30, 2012, issue of the *American Journal of Clinical Nutrition*, involving a total of 9,514 women, both Chinese and American, and confirming that "despite large differences in soy isoflavone intake by country, isoflavone consumption was inversely associated with recurrence among both American and Chinese women." Researchers concluded in this pooled analysis that women who ate roughly 10 mg of isoflavones a day had a "statistically relevant protection against recurrence."

*Soy foods listed from least to most processed*

*Soybeans* are tasty whether eaten as a high-protein main course, or thrown into a soup, casserole, or salad. They are quite mild when cooked properly, with a texture that holds up nicely in all types of recipes.

*Edamame (edda-mah-may)* are young, green, whole soybeans. They are typically left in the pod for cooking, by boiling or steaming, and then are traditionally topped with sea salt.

*Tempeh (tem-pay, and I've heard the accent on either syllable)* is a fermented soy product made with soybeans and grain. It has a dense, chewy, toothsome texture that is perfect for sandwiches or crumbled into other dishes, and it makes a tasty sloppy joe.

*Miso (mee-so)* is a scrumptious, salty, and nutritious condiment in paste form that is made by placing soybeans, grain, and salt in a fermenting culture. It adds umami (pleasant, rich flavor) to soups, sauces, dressings, and marinades. There are quite a few different kinds of miso, from mellow to super-strong, using different kinds of grains. I love to stir a tablespoon of miso into a cup of water for a quick and delicious cuppa broth. To make a more filling snack, I often toss in a tablespoon of chia seeds, which will quickly absorb the liquid and turn the broth into a warm, savory pudding sort of thing.

*Tofu* (soybean curd) is a spongy and sort of cheesy-textured food that's made by curdling and pressing fresh hot soymilk. There are quite a few different kinds, and they are available in larger (and some smaller) grocery stores. From softest to firmest: *Silken tofu* is creamy and very soft and is great for making your own "creamy" dressings (like mayo), soups (like cream-of-whatever), and desserts (like "cheesecake"). It blends like a champ. It often comes in an aseptic pack and stores well in the pantry. *Soft tofu* is slightly firmer and is also good in blended soups.

*Firm and extra-firm tofu* are great for cubing and tossing into stir fries, soups, salads, or made into "kind of cheesy-like" foods like ricotta or feta substitutes. *Sprouted soybean tofu* is produced in such a way to make the final product more digestible.

*Soy flour* is made with soybeans that have been roasted prior to grinding.

It's found in many baked goods and can be used in home baking as well, although, because it doesn't have gluten, it should be mixed with other flours that *do* have gluten, using only small ratios of the soy flour. If the end product will be a yeast bread, you can only substitute up to 15% soy flour, and if not yeast-based, you can substitute up to a quarter of it. This substitution will increase the nutrition and protein content of the end product.

*Soy milk* is the rich liquid that is extracted from soybeans, high in protein and low in saturated fat. It can be substituted one-for-one with dairy milk in recipes. It is fortified just as dairy milk is. I should note here that in the same way that fruit juices are not as nutritious as the whole fiber-rich fruit they used to occupy, so with soymilk. It's good, and it's tasty, but don't drink it all day in place of water; use in moderation, or never. I only buy it on those rare occasions when I can't find another plain nut or grain milk.

*Texturized Vegetable Protein (TVP) and Texturized Soy Protein (TSP)* are highly-processed soy products that should pretty much be avoided unless organic, and then only occasionally. If it isn't organic, which would include 98% of the TVP/TSP produced, it has been created with the use of hexane, some sort of a gasoline-related chemical, which is something that I personally have no interest in putting in my mouth, now or ever. How they pulled off that being legal is beyond me, and beyond the scope of this book, but: Yowza.

Manufacturing this stuff from (defatted soy flour) is a complex process that starts with the use of high heat and a caustic alkaline solution to pull out the protein. It is then mixed with an acid solution to again pull out the protein, then dipped once more, this time in an alkaline solution, and finally sprayed out and dried at extremely high temps. It is often spun into protein fibers or extruded into meaty-looking shapes. I have found only one brand at my health food store that is organic: Soy Curls. I use it for small things like a bacony-bits type condiment I make (and use very sparingly). Otherwise, my best advice is to stay away from TVP and TSP. Blech.

### *The worst of the worst: soy protein isolates and concentrates*

*Soy protein isolates (SPIs) and soy protein concentrates (SPCs)* are the most highly-processed soy foods, also made from defatted soy flour from which most of the carbs and fats have been chemically stripped away. This is a by-product (actually, a waste product) of the gigantic soybean oil industry and as such is ridiculously cheap for food manufacturers to purchase as a food ingredient, which is why it is being added to just about every "high protein" food being sold to satisfy the current media craze, the high protein diet, including, but not limited to high protein shake mixes (yup, even the ones that say "natural"), protein bars (yup, even the ones that say "natural"), high protein cereals (well, you know what I'm gonna say here), and most (but not all) fake-meaty analogs, veggie burgers, hotdogs, and meaty crumbles, like those ubiquitous green packages in your local supermarket freezer case. Do not eat these. Ever. And don't let anyone you love eat 'em either, even if they have never had cancer!

It is not tricky to get adequate protein on a plan that supports breast cancer nutrition, and these highly processed products are best avoided completely. While we have plenty of research available on the safety of whole (or near-whole) soy foods, especially the fermented products, we know nothing about these super-high protein, super-processed-with-ridiculous-chemicals foods and food additives and how they affect our hormonal systems.

I avoid any food that lists soy protein isolate as an ingredient, in any amount, and will do so until I have evidence that this common-sense approach to the food we eat is not warranted. Read your labels, as it is hidden in many, many foods, including cereals, protein shakes, and protein bars.

For more information about the history of soy and chemical solvents being used in the production of protein-enriched products, please check out the website for the Cornucopia Institute. They have some fairly extensive discussions on chemical solvents used in everyday processed foods along with a listing of companies that have been checked out and are truly natural.

### Do not take soy supplements

Many have been led to believe that, when it comes to taking a nutritional supplement, if the small amount found in food is good, then more must be even better. However, not only is there absolutely no evidence to suggest that soy isoflavone or genistein supplements are beneficial to breast cancer survivors, there is much that suggests that supplementation may be detrimental. For that reason, the medical community advises not to use them. (And remember, the highest quality nutrition is always found in its original packaging. With love from Momma Nature.)

### THE BOTTOM LINE

Eat a serving of organic soy three to five times a week, from whole, organically grown and processed soybeans, including the fermented products tempeh and miso. Avoid more processed forms such as soy milk, and eliminate soy protein isolate completely from your diet, looking for hidden sources in common processed foods such as protein drinks and cereals. Do not use soy supplements.

# 31. DRINK GREEN TEA, FILTERED WATER, AND NON-DAIRY MILK

The three main varieties of non-herbal tea—green, black, and oolong—all come from the same evergreen tree that grows up to 30 feet high in the wild but is pruned to a manageable size of about three feet for farm production. Camellia sinensis is the plant from which all teas originate and is primarily grown in China.

The undeniable champion of healthy tea is green, which is made from unfermented tea leaves, and of the three varieties has the most powerful concentration of the phytonutrient ECGC.

Over 90 different studies of bioavailability have shown that our plasma concentrations of ECGC peak about 1½ to 2½ hours after drinking it and that it is pretty much gone in nine hours. Animal studies have also shown that the tea polyphenols absorbed in the gastric tract are widely distributed to other organs. The antioxidant ability of our bodies increases, along with other biomarkers of DNA oxidative damage, which, as we now know, is a precursor to cancer mutation.

ECGC shuts down the main relay station from which growth factors for cancer send their messages. Referred to as tyrosine kinase receptors, they are essential for transmitting the messages sent by these growth factors. ECGCs are also triggers of cancer cell death and cell cycle arrest. Recent human studies strongly suggest that green tea may indeed reduce the risk of all cancers, including breast cancer.

A summary report of observational studies completed in 2012 in the journal *Functional Foods in Health and Disease* concluded that there is strong evidence that higher green tea consumption is associated with a decrease in the risk of breast cancers. The authors of the report added that this is supported by strong evidence of the tumor-inhibitory effects of green tea in animal studies as well as in vitro and in vivo experiments.

Another Japanese study reported that women (particularly those with early stage, primary cancers) consuming at least three cups of green tea a day had 57% fewer relapses than those drinking less.

Beliveau and Gingras wrote in the journal *Lancet* that three four-ounce cups of green tea was a sufficient amount to block most of the receptors that would allow cancer to invade neighboring cells; these same receptors also serve to stimulate blood vessels that feed growing tumors.

*Fat loss and bone mineral density*

Green tea not only supports our anti-breast cancer agenda, but our fat loss goals as well, working to promote the loss of fat that accumulates in the tissues lining the abdominal cavity and associated with metabolic syndromes. A study published in the January 2005 *American Journal of Clinical Nutrition* reported that men drinking 690 mg of green tea catechins (those are the potent flavonoids in green tea, including ECGC) for 12 weeks lost weight and body fat, as well as realizing a significant drop in LDL cholesterol and free radicals. Green tea is also useful for maintaining a healthy bone mineral density.

*How to buy it*

Organic loose-leaf green tea is far superior to tea bags when it comes to obtaining the highest quality catechins. Most of the packaged tea found in grocery (and even health food) stores is made with the powdery "fannings and dust" from the tea production process and are low quality teas at best. The phytonutrient substances in green tea will degrade with air and light, and will even seep into the tea bags they are stored in, over time.

My very favorite variety is gunpowder green tea, purchased loose and made with whole-leaf tea that has been withered, steamed, rolled into little pellets, and dried. When the leaves later come in contact with water they unfurl to their original size, most of the ECGC intact. On the road, I use a metal or cloth tea infuser to brew my tea, and a beautiful ceramic infuser at home. I will often eat some of the tea leaves for added benefit.

I purchase bulk organic green tea at great prices from Frontier Natural Products Co-op (online) through a local buying club I have been a member of for a number of years. Even without the discount provided through the buying club, this is a cost-effective way to purchase green tea, as a one-pound package of tea lasts a good long time—only a scant teaspoonful is used per cup.

*Other ways to use green tea—and more synergy coming your way*

You can add a little ginger juice to your tea, or lemon, which unlocks bioavailability through the polyphenol synergy we are beginning to know and love so well. You can make green tea chai by gently brewing tea in nut-milk and adding a dash of black pepper, cinnamon, allspice, ginger, and cardamom. You could also brew it in cool water for 20 to 30 minutes and add to other recipes instead of water or broth. You can cook soba (buckwheat) or other noodles in it.

In 2012, researchers at Rutgers University published a study in the journal *Food and Function* in which the phytochemical quercetin (found in many fruits and vegetables, especially apples with the skin on) increased the bioavailability and quadrupled cellular absorption of green tea's anti-cancer component, ECGC, which sounded like a perfect excuse to poach apples in green tea. So I did. It was good.

One other way to integrate the great phytonutrients of green tea into your system is by tossing spent tea leaves right into your food, including smoothies, salads, dressings, soups, and casseroles.

*Black tea may promote breast cancer*

A meta-analysis of the research available on black tea in relation to breast cancer risk was reported in the journal *Carcinogenesis* in July, 2006. Researchers Sun, Yuan, and Yu concluded that there was a modest increase in breast cancer risk associated with consuming black tea and that it may have a promotional effect on later stage breast cancer. Black tea is made from the same leaves as green tea, but the processing is very different, involving a fermentation or oxidation of the leaves.

Although green tea is enjoying resurgence, black tea is still highly popular. You will find it in Earl Grey and other English (or Irish) breakfast and afternoon teas. Black tea is also the variety traditionally used in making chai. While an occasional cup of black tea or chai is unlikely to cause great harm, it is my intention to steer clear of things that may promote breast cancer.

*Milk products*

As a former dairy milk aficionada, I was delighted to discover that there are a wide variety of non-dairy milks to choose from when making this particular dietary changeover, and they are fairly easy to make yourself, as well. Two of the most common homemade milks are almond and cashew, made with raw nuts, clean water, and a blender. The packaged milks are fortified just as dairy milk is.

I don't drink soy milk by the glass, only because a half cupful constitutes one serving, and on a diet that is well-managed for soy consumption it's simply too easy to drink more than I really need in my diet. It also isn't a whole soy food, which is the best source of the soy isoflavones I am looking for.

### Good, clean water

We require water to keep all of our bodily processes humming along. I do keep water nearby and take sips all day long. Your body only uses a little at a time and doesn't store vast useable reserves like a camel, so drinking a gigantic glass of water all at once probably isn't your best strategy.

So: Drink water all day, especially if you are thirsty. I really don't force myself to drink a certain amount, but I do pay attention to my body's needs and make sure to hydrate properly. You will be eating a lot of fruits and veggies, and there's water in those, as well. Our bodies have a way of asking for water when they need it. We simply need to listen.

Find out whether your local water supply is clean, and if not, make sure that you filter the water you drink and cook with. If you can't afford a whole-house filtration system, you can cheaply and easily invest in a filtered pitcher to sit on the kitchen counter.

Don't drink out of bottles made with BPAs, which are plausible estrogen-disruptors, and most certainly don't drink bottled water that has been sitting in a car in the sun for any length of time, getting hot and leaching nasty chemicals into it, and last but not least, do not drink out of a hose that's been sitting around in your yard all day filled with water and bacteria and who-on-earth-knows-what kind of nasty and disgusting carcinogenic petrochemicals.

### THE BOTTOM LINE

There's more than one way to hydrate! Drink four small cups of green tea daily, from good quality whole leaf green tea, spaced evenly through the day. Milk lovers can either make or buy delicious nut and seed milks for drinking and cooking. Drink good, clean water when you are thirsty and make it into delicious, apigenin-rich, and calming chamomile tea; and finally, drink black tea only occasionally.

# 32. DRINK BETWEEN ZERO AND ONE
## SERVING OF ALCOHOL A WEEK

Alcohol consumption has been correlated with cancer risk in the research community for at least 20 years. It was reported in the *Journal of the American Medical Association* that even low, regular use of alcohol increases the risk, generally speaking, of dying of cancer. A meta-analysis completed in 1994 confirmed the existence of a strong relationship between alcohol and breast cancer, which was again confirmed in 2013 by Jin *et al.*

These studies, however, were relevant to the risk of primary breast cancer, and not to recurrence, which is where our primary interest lies. It was hypothesized at the time that alcohol's influence on our prognosis would have something to do with how it increases estrogen metabolism and raises estrogen levels, particularly among postmenopausal women, but none of the studies, until recently, had a large sample size, which was a concern.

The After Breast Cancer Pooling Project (ABCPP) sought to remedy that concern, gathering data on 9,329 breast cancer survivors in the United States. The ABCPP showed that (compared to non-drinkers) regular consumption of more than a half a drink a day was associated with an approximate 20% increase in the relative risk of recurrence; several other large studies confirm these findings. A half a drink is defined as 2.5 ounces of wine, 6 ounces of beer, or .75 ounces of liquor.

Given that this behavior is simple to modify, I didn't have great difficulty cutting alcohol out of my life almost completely, with the exception of a truly occasional glass of wine on special occasions. I even happily modified a ritual that used to involve drinking alcohol with my dad: Every Wednesday in the summer the two of us enjoy Martini Night, and have, for some time. We sit on the deck overlooking a little lake and talk, and I help him finish his crossword puzzles, and we solve the great philosophical issues of our life and times, and also drink martinis.

Even though I still hang out with him every Wednesday night in the summer, and even though I still am required in my heart of hearts to call it Martini Night, my martini has become a glass of sparkling water with lemon, to which I blissfully add an occasional teaspoon of vodka.

And I'm okay with that.

## THE BOTTOM LINE

While an occasional serving of alcohol is acceptable, it's time to say goodbye to our regular drinking days, consuming no more than one drink each week for what researchers advise will bring maximum long-term results.

# 33. AVOID KNOWN ENVIRONMENTAL HAZARDS TO YOUR BREAST HEALTH

In 2011, the National Academy of Sciences (NAS) undertook the task of reviewing the current evidence on breast cancer risk and the environment. They concluded in their extensive report that there are a few general areas under our control that have been shown to have an impact on breast cancer risk.

They advise that we can avoid unnecessary medical radiation, we can avoid combination hormone therapy unless medically appropriate, we can avoid active and passive smoking, we can take appropriate dietary and exercise measures, we can eliminate or carefully restrict the use of alcohol, we can consider the use of anti-hormone medication such as Tamoxifen or aromatase inhibitors if we are high risk (which we are), and finally, we can limit or eliminate workplace, consumer, and environmental exposure to dangerous and toxic chemicals that the NAS considers highly likely contributors to breast cancer.

Throughout this book, I have often referred to scientific research and discussed percentages, statistics, and risk factors as though it were possible to disentangle one risk factor—or one positive step we can take— from the complicated biological system that is our bodies, and in doing so discuss various risks completely in isolation from each other, which we know just isn't possible.

*Why isn't there a simple recurrence calculation?*

Wouldn't it be incredible if we could perform this simple calculation: My tumor's genomic analysis came back with an $x\%$ chance of recurrence, so I eat broccoli (odds improvement = $b\%$), begin an exercise program ($+e\%$), maintain a healthy weight (+w%), add flaxseed to my daily menu (+f%), eat blueberries (+bl%), use turmeric and black pepper (+t%+p%), and limit my alcohol to one glass of wine a week at most (+a%), and, based on the simple math, I now have an exact r% chance of recurrence.

Sigh. I really wish it worked that way, but there is no such formula to be conjured up. Instead, the behaviors we exhibit, those that help and those that hinder our health, all roll around inside us, bumping into each other, gaining energy and strength from each other whether for good or evil, and interacting in mysterious, synergistic ways that we really can't put numbers on. Another heavy sigh.

But that's okay, it really is. You are gaining a great understanding of how this ol' bod of yours works, and you are simply going to do as much as you can, as soon as you are able, to give yourself a fighting chance to join me in becoming an old lady one of these days. Some of the things we will do, such as a whole foods, plant-based anti-breast cancer diet and the daily exercise we've added to our lives, add to the positive synergy bumping around in there, and some take away from it. To follow is a discussion of the negative things that will diminish our chances of being cancer-free old women some day, according to the NAS report.

*Cigarettes and chemicals*

We need to avoid first-, second-, and third-hand smoke. Among the suspect chemicals the NAS looked at, the evidence for an association with breast cancer risk was clearest for ethylene oxide, as well as benzene and 1,3-butadiene. One sure way to expose yourself to these chemicals is through active or passive smoking. These same three carcinogenic chemicals that are found in cigarette smoke are used in numerous industrial and medical applications.

For example, benzene is added to fuel and occurs naturally in crude oil, which makes vehicle emissions at gas stations or on the farm a common source of exposure. Another chemical of special concern to the NAS is bisphenol-A, or BPA, which is still commonly used as a plastic hardener in many containers used for storing food or water.

To minimize your contact with BPA, don't microwave food in plastic containers and don't use water bottles that are old or scratched. Instead, use glass in the microwave and buy a metal bottle that is not lined with plastic (many are). One study even found that people's BPA levels were reduced simply by reducing the amount of pre-packaged and canned foods consumed. (Canned tomato products are a particular offender due to their acid content.)

One study, completed by the Silent Spring Institute, found that the average indoor air sample contained 19 different estrogen-disrupting chemicals and 27 different pesticides. We can do a great deal to eliminate this toxic environment by safely disposing of all the products stored in our homes that we use for cleaning or pest management and by replacing them with either purchased products that are gentle on the environment (and us) or by making them ourselves from simple and inexpensive ingredients.

### Norwex cleaning cloths are amazing

I am a huge fan of Norwex cleaning cloths, used not only to clean but also to disinfect with nothing more than water. They're pretty amazing, and you must believe me when I say I am pretty close to being the most skeptical person in the world when it comes to this kind of thing. There are similar products that work "okay," and imitators, for sure, but there's only one real deal. And it's a woman-owned company for good measure. (No, I don't own stock in Norwex, but I wish I did!)

### Dietary supplements

Make sure you talk to your oncologist or nutritionist about any supplements you may think you want to use, especially for weight loss or control of menopausal symptoms, as they possibly contain hormonally active ingredients that will work against your antiestrogen life strategy.

Dr. T. Colin Campbell, in his amazing book, *Whole*, has written extensively on this topic, providing detailed information on why it is generally a bad idea to get nutrients from supplements that have been divorced from their source. (Great book. Read it when things slow down.)

It is vital that you work closely with your doctor or nutritionist to make sure that you are getting all of the essentials through your diet, or to begin supplementation if not.

### Cosmetics

The NAS also expressed concern about many cosmetics, especially those marketed to "turn back the hands of time," as they are likely to have hormonally active ingredients. Ridiculous loopholes in FDA regulations (gigantic enough to drive a truck through) allow companies in the United States that manufacture cosmetics and personal care products the opportunity to put just about anything they want in their products with little or no concern for whether they are carcinogenic. Here's just some of the toxic crap that's allowed, and how each may impact you on your journey to health:

## Phthalates

Phthalates are endocrine disruptors found most commonly in nail polish and synthetic fragrances (as the perfume itself, or as an ingredient). Regular exposure to phthalates has been linked to early onset of puberty and is a likely risk factor for breast cancer. Some of these chemicals have been found to act as weak estrogens in vitro.

## 1,4-dioxane

1,4-dioxane makes up the bubbles in your bubble bath (and your children's bubble bath, too). It is also in shampoo, body wash, and other foaming, bubbling products.

## Parabens

Parabens are widely used as cosmetic antifungal agents and are found in lotions, shampoos, cosmetics, and deodorants. They have been widely identified in biopsy samples of breast cancer tumors and are found in many incarnations at the grocery store. Look for the word "paraben" as a part of the ingredient listed, such as methylparaben.

## Ethylene oxide

Ethylene oxide is found in fragrances and is an ingredient in most mass-marketed shampoos. It is a known human carcinogen according to the National Toxicology Program (NTP) and is known to cause mammary cancer in mice. It is also found in dry-cleaning solution.

## Polycrylic aromatic hydrocarbons (PAHs)

Polycrylic aromatic hydrocarbons (PAHs) are found naturally in gas and oil and can be found in products made with coal tar, often used for psoriasis concoctions. They may increase breast cancer risk.

## Placental extract

Placental extract comes from either human or animal placentas and is used most often in products marketed to African American women. The NTP has identified the progesterone in this ingredient as a reasonably anticipated carcinogen.

### Deodorant, sunscreen, and cosmetics

Aluminum is found in deodorants. It mimics estrogen and has the ability to damage DNA. I'm not going to blow smoke up your skirt. There aren't any studies showing a direct link between aluminum and breast cancer, but researchers have found a concentration of aluminum in the same areas where most primary breast cancer tumors are found. Research has shown that up to 60% of all breast tumors are found in the area of the breast nearest the underarm.

Of course, none of this proves causation, and I know scientific inquiry well enough to know that this one is sketchy, but it *does* suggest that women who have already proven that they are more likely to be diagnosed with breast cancer might best steer clear of it. Why take the chance when there are so many other truly natural options that work just as well?

Sunscreens have been found to have chemical components that exert significant estrogenic activity in laboratory experiments, and these chemicals are showing up in humans, as well.

Mammary carcinogens have been found in many cosmetics, including those listed above, as well as 1,3-butadiene. That's the same crap you breathe in from active and passive smoking, and it's also found in shaving cream, hair products, and some high-SPF sunscreens. Benzene comes from the fumes you breathe in at the gas station, and are also found in nail polish by way of toluene. BPA is found in many cosmetic packaging materials; petrolatum is found in petroleum jelly, lipstick, baby lotion, and oils, and urethane is found in hair mousse, gel, hairspray, sunscreen, nail polish, mascara, and foundation.

## THE BOTTOM LINE

Protect yourself from this chemical onslaught by avoiding most mass-marketed cosmetics, nail polishes, hair care products, and deodorants that contain these harmful carcinogens. Safe alternatives for all of these products, including sunscreen, exist! It's also a good idea to air out your dry-cleaned clothes (outside the plastic covering) before returning them to the closet. "Outgassing" new furniture in fresh air for a few days (at a minimum) is also a practical idea; you might even consider purchasing furniture, carpet and rugs that have not been sprayed with flame-retardants and other carcinogenic chemicals.

# 34. STOP COUNTING CALORIES
## AND OTHER USEFUL INFORMATION:
## A SUMMARY

I wasted a fair number of otherwise perfectly wonderful years obsessing over how many calories I put into my mouth, somewhat (but not completely) oblivious to the vastly more important task of paying attention to the quality of the food that I ate.

Am I saying that calories don't matter? Well, of course not! If I put too many empty, nutritionless calories into my body, I am going to have to store them somewhere. However, the simple truth of the matter is that we have bigger fish to fry than that. (Hmmm, I believe I need to invest in a new metaphoric cliché, because there is no fish on the menu, and I wouldn't be frying it up if it was.)

And so, as we begin to change the overall paradigm of our lives, we begin to see all of the things we pay attention to in a compelling new light, and we learn to count the things that really do matter. I feel as though I have reached the place where I've given you all the science you could possibly manage to digest, and possibly more: So let me cut to the chase.

*Track things that really matter*

Breast cancer survivors are now being advised to aim for *35 to 40 grams of fiber a day*, from whole grains, vegetables, fruits, and beans. This would translate into *four to six servings of whole grains, one to two servings of beans or legumes*, and *nine servings of fruits and veggies a day, two of which are crucifers*, with an emphasis on choosing a minimum of *three different colors* each day for maximum nutrient values.

Let's keep track of the *four small cups of green tea*, spread equally through-out the day, that will not only serve up the powerful catechin ECGC but will keep our metabolism in overdrive, and let's make sure we include *three tablespoons of freshly-ground flaxseed* on our daily menu.

And let's also track the exercise we engage in on a weekly basis, so we get *three to five hours of moderate exercise* each week that includes some basic resistance and strength.

## *Focus on "the nature and quality" of your food*

Dr. Neal Barnard's advice to cancer survivors also focuses on the nature and quality of the food consumed rather than the number of calories. His recommendations, which are in line with those of the breast cancer nutri-tionist I have on my team, call for a diet that is designed around 55-75% complex carbohydrates, 10-15% protein, and 10-20% healthy fats, which he suggests ought to account for no more than 35 grams a day. (My nutrition-ist goes up to 25% on the healthy fats.)

## *Eat organic food when it is possible and practical*

I will not make a big speech here. I just want to say, simply, that it's great to eat organic as often as is available and as often as your budget allows. One of our most important jobs as breast cancer survivors is to avoid as many carcinogens, hormone disruptors, and toxins as we possibly can, which will give us a leg-up at avoiding recurrence, and one of the biggest ways we can avoid carcinogens (along with our daily-use personal and hygiene products) is by eating organic food.

Organic food is grown without the assistance of chemical pesticides, fer-tilizers, biotechnology, growth hormones, or irradiation. Not only does or-ganic farming promote sustainable agriculture, but it also conserves re-sources and reduces water pollution. Research is still out as to whether or-ganic food in and of itself has more nutrients than non-organic, but the point that must be made here is in regard to the toxic load of non-organic food.

If you don't have fresh organic produce available to you, or your budget doesn't allow it, the rule of thumb is that it is still better for you to eat the fruits and veggies in front of you, no matter the source, than to skip them entirely. Eat your veggies and fruit!

*The Dirty Dozen and the Clean Fifteen*

One of the best tools we have is ongoing analysis performed by the Environmental Working Group (EWG), an organization that looks at data gathered by USDA and FDA scientists each year and publishes the *Shopper's Guide to Pesticides in Produce*, a listing of common fruits and veggies that carry the lowest and highest toxic loads.

This information is translated into the Dirty Dozen and Clean Fifteen, which are handy guides of fruits and vegetables that are generally to be avoided, unless organic, and those that are generally safe. Bear in mind that the fruits and veggies being analyzed are washed extremely well prior to being sampled, and if they are typically eaten without skins (like bananas, pineapples, and oranges), they are removed prior to testing. To repeat: The produce is washed thoroughly *before* testing for pesticides. That means if a fruit or vegetable is listed as having a heavy pesticide load, it will be there after you wash it. And if you don't wash it, you are really asking for trouble.

The 2013 Dirty Dozen are apples (almost always at the top of the "don't eat unless organic most of the time" list), strawberries, grapes, celery, peaches, spinach, sweet bell peppers, imported nectarines, cucumbers, potatoes, cherry tomatoes, and hot peppers. This list was expanded to highlight two crops, domestically grown summer squash and leafy greens, specifically kale and collard greens. These two crops were not in the top 12 in *quantity* of pesticide load, but were commonly contaminated with pesticides that are exceptionally dangerous to the human nervous system.

Those fruits and vegetables with the least pesticide load in 2013 consists of corn, onions, pineapples, avocados, cabbage, frozen sweet peas, papayas, mangoes, asparagus, eggplant, kiwi, grapefruit, cantaloupe, sweet potatoes, and mushrooms.

*Something that is "vegan" is not necessarily "good for you"*

There are plenty of vegans who do not obtain the nutrients that are required by a healthy adult. There are plenty of ingredients that are vegan but are not healthy. There are plenty of vegan foods that are loaded with sugar, fat, refined grains, and/or other ingredients that you do not want to put in your mouth, including many processed and prepared foods, cookies, snacks, and desserts, most packaged food in grocery stores, and just about anything that has an advertising budget. (Oreos are vegan.) So this isn't just about being a vegan.

Healthy food isn't expensive, or at least doesn't have to be, especially if you are willing to spend a little extra time in the kitchen and to learn about new, whole food ingredients. The important thing is to make most of your food choices from whole, nutritious, plant-based foods.

*A food that is "organic" is not necessarily "good for you"*

Along the same line of reasoning, not all organic food is going to be appropriate for our very specific nutritional requirements, including organic sugar, organic white flour, and organic fats. Examples of organic foods that don't meet our needs would be organic corn chips fried in organic canola oil, high-fat and high-sugar organic desserts, and organic fruit juices.

*Goal food groups and serving sizes for each*

It might seem to you that there just aren't enough hours in the day for you to eat all of the servings of whole grains, fresh fruits, and vegetables that the experts are advising, so let's take a look at the actual size of various servings, in the hope that it'll help put to things in perspective.

My daily smoothie has one cup of leafy greens, a half a cup of crucifers, and a cup of fruit in it, and I typically eat one very large salad at another meal, which pretty much covers the rest of it. Here are serving sizes for various whole foods:

*Vegetables: 6 or more servings a day (2 of which are crucifers)*
½ cup of cooked veggies or 1 cup of raw veggies

*Fruits: 3 servings a day*
1 small piece of whole fruit
½ cup of cooked or chopped fresh fruit or ¼ cup of dried fruit

*Legumes: 1-3 servings a day*
½ cup of cooked beans, lentils, or other legumes
¼ cup of low-fat bean spread
1 cup of non-dairy milk
3 ounces of tofu, tempeh, seitan, or meat alternative

*Whole grains and pastas: 4-6 servings a day*
½ cup of cooked whole grain
1 ounce of dry pasta, rice or dry grain
1 slice of bread or ½ of a pita bread or tortilla

1 small muffin (one ounce) or 1 cup of ready-to-eat cereal

*Freshly-ground flaxseed: 1-3 servings a day*
1 tablespoon

*Green tea: 4 servings a day*
1 cup of fresh-brewed, whole leaf tea (7-8 ounces)

## *Fiber goal*

It bears repeating that we are aiming for *35 to 40 grams of fiber a day*. The servings of food listed above should get you to this goal, but it might be interesting to track your fiber with one of the online nutrition analyzers, such as can be found at the NutritionData or Livestrong websites, just to get a feel for it.

## *Fat goal*

A high-fat diet is highly associated with increased risk of recurrence. The nutritionist I work with advises that I keep my fat intake to *no more than 25% of total calories, which would break down to 26-30 grams of fat a day*. This would allow for a small amount of added fat from extra virgin olive oil; fat grams consumed would be interesting to track, as well, at least while making the transition to a new whole foods plant-based diet.

## *Saturated fat goal*

Most of the time, aim for zero grams of saturated fat. It is mainly obtained in our diets as fat from animal sources but will also come from coconut oil, palm kernel oil, and cocoa butter, fats that are hard at room temperature.

## *THE BOTTOM LINE*

Follow the outlined recommendations in this chapter, put together for our benefit by nutritionists, doctors, and researchers who know what they are talking about, to maximize vitality and good health.

# PHASE THREE: THE LOVE

Adding layers of depth to life,
embracing the new normal,
and getting more cowbell!

*"Wrap yourself in the armor of love and take courage."*

~ My friend Sheila, to me

# 35. EVALUATE ALL RELATIONSHIPS

The initial traumatic shock and emotional upheaval of diagnosis very quickly give way to the business (and busy-ness) of treatment and recovery. We are constantly on the road, filling out never-ending paperwork, undergoing tests, and talking on the telephone. We keep appointments with a dizzying array of doctors and specialists. We undergo surgery and subsequent recovery and endure the unrelenting grind of day after day in radiation treatments.

We are poked, prodded, stripped down to the waist, looked at, palpated, and sometimes discussed as though we weren't sitting right there. It is no small wonder that so many of us succumb to feelings of hopelessness or depression: Our lives, changed forever in a dramatic nanosecond, now seem, at times, completely out-of-our-control.

I have been truly blessed with an extensive circle of friends, near and far, old and new, who were (and continue to be) good medicine not just for my heart, but for my health, as I faced and learned how to cope with the new set of challenges and realities immediately presenting themselves. My hubby, Mike, stood by my side as often as I needed him to.

(I must confess to being more than a little independent and self-reliant, so I think it's fair to say that he was sometimes at a loss for exactly what to do for me. Nonetheless, when I needed him, there he was, quiet and steady, and I was glad for that.)

Research has confirmed what I know deep inside: Interpersonal relationships play a huge role in recovery, and a woman whose marriage is in discord will suffer the negative physical consequences of this chronic stress. It seems clear that while a breast cancer diagnosis doesn't cause problems in a marriage, it certainly will have the effect of shining a light in the dark and ugly corners of an unhappy one.

Further, science tells us that cardiovascular, endocrine, and immune re-

159

sponses are impaired in people in unhappy marriages. For that reason, it came as no great surprise that Ohio State University researchers recently concluded that marital distress is not only associated with worse psychological outcomes for breast cancer survivors, but that women in unhappy marriages also had poorer overall health and suffered a decline in physical activity after diagnosis. Their data also showed that recovery was slower for those who were additionally coping with marital problems.

Even the quality of familial support systems has been shown to exert a tremendous influence on our survival. A report published in the journal *Breast Cancer* found that, among 4,530 women followed, those experiencing what they referred to as a "high social strain," and with a large number of generally unsupportive relatives, had a higher mortality rate across the board, and not just for breast cancer survivors.

The results of an observational study at UCLA's School of Medicine concurred: Negative social interactions can quite easily be linked to increased inflammation, a pro-cancer agent. The researchers went on to say that people who surround themselves with other upbeat, happy people may be less susceptible to diseases that are associated with the inflammatory process.

> Research has confirmed what I know deep inside: Interpersonal relationships play a huge role in recovery, and a woman whose marriage is in discord will suffer the negative physical consequences of this chronic stress.

Women who are dealing with a breast cancer diagnosis absolutely must surround themselves with high-quality relationships that serve to bolster them up. A bad marriage, or other unhealthy emotional relationships, undermines the way we approach the world, how we feel about ourselves, and ultimately, our overall health and well-being.

A breast cancer diagnosis is a touchstone moment in our lives; for me, my life is easily divided into Before Breast Cancer and After Breast Cancer. It has changed me at the very deepest core of who I am. I came out the other side stronger, more confident, ready to take on the world, way less willing to waste my time, and a thousand percent more willing to let things go that do not mean something to me, whether a "thing" in my house or a relationship that is unhealthy. (I am also way more cranky when pushed a little too far. Don't test me.)

There's something about facing the possibility of my own death that sharpened my awareness that life is precious, and I have even less desire to spend time with people who don't bring light and joy into my life, or to do things that I really don't enjoy doing, or to engage in conversations or debates that serve no purpose. (Unless, of course, I have to. I really can put on my big girl panties when I need to, and I know you can too.)

## THE BOTTOM LINE

Take this opportunity to evaluate all of the relationships in your life, all of the things and places and people you fill your day with, and when you find that something just isn't working, commit to doing the work that will make it better. Or realize that it's simply time to move on. Because we know that life is precious. And it's time to make it really count.

# 36. JOIN A SUPPORT GROUP (OR NOT)

If you've recently been diagnosed with breast cancer, chances are pretty good that you are still reeling with the news, as I was in the first weeks. Mike, bless his heart, was not fully able to listen to me talk about the fears that were pounding through my head much of the day and into the night in those first wobbly weeks and months.

So many of the initial questions I had were not necessarily related to the science of my experience but were about the heart and soul of it. I desperately needed to talk to someone, to other women who were also on this same frightening path.

Because I am an open and avid user of social networking, I was almost immediately connected to a small group of women, friends of friends, who generously entered into long-distance conversations that I am 100% certain kept me from losing my mind. I also contacted the local Gilda's Club chapter, in Grand Rapids, Michigan, and spent many hours there between appointments, mainly in the warm and comfy library, reading books, meditating, or sometimes, just letting go with a good cry.

If I had not had these outlets, I believe that I would have searched for a support group. There are some points to consider when deciding whether to pursue this particular therapeutic support; a formal breast cancer group may or may not be for you. I informally polled a few women who had experienced a support group to find out what parts of it worked and what parts didn't.

*What worked for them? Here's what they said.*

They said that there's no one who gets what we are going through and what we are dealing with as well as another woman who has been in our shoes; that other survivors really get it and get where we are coming from.

163

That there seems to come a time when our friends and family don't want to talk about breast cancer anymore (like we often do, and often need to); that our friends and families may reach their limit on this topic of conversation, and they may reach that limit way sooner than we need it to be, because this is a topic of almost never-ending interest to many of us.

That there are blessings and gifts to be found in sharing our experience; that others who are walking our path can tell us about their own positive experiences, helping us to have hope for the future; that our sisters can also help us to celebrate victories that may seem insignificant to others.

That other survivors will be a wealth of information on life hacks, tricks of the trade, and coping mechanisms for everything from nausea to trying to feel beautiful again; that if we stay in a group long-term, we will someday be able to help a new survivor as we are now being helped.

That positive lifestyle changes are more successful when we have a group to report back to; that breast cancer survivors in a local support group will be able to give us information about local resources.

That there is great comfort to be found when we can say something that for once needs no further definition, translation, or explanation.

And simply, that there is friendship to be found in a support group.

*And what didn't work for them?*

They said that, just like any group, if not well-facilitated, it can be disorganized or could even be taken over by big personalities; that if a woman is quiet, she may not be heard.

That it is possible for us to hear things that are terrifying and sad at a time in our journeys when that is just too much to handle.

That some support groups may be too therapeutic, or not therapeutic enough, for our needs; that the nature of what we are experiencing is such that we are likely to become deeply bonded with women who will lose their lives to breast cancer. (That's a big one for me. Really big.)

## THE BOTTOM LINE

It's a good idea to talk to the sponsor of the group to get more detail about how her particular group functions, as there is a great deal of diversity. Some groups just have interesting speakers, or once-a-month get-togethers for a meal and conversation. Check it out before you commit by attending at least one meeting, to get the feel of the group and to see if it's a good fit. If it doesn't feel right, trust your instincts.

A support group may be just what you need. Or not.

# 37. SMILE, LAUGH, AND PLAY, EVERY DAMN DAY

There are times when I am having such a particularly difficult day, when my chest is tight and I'm so emotionally plugged up that even my go-to breathing exercises don't work. It's then that my inclination is to do absolutely nothing but sit somewhere like a lump. Bah! When I'm in that place, I have a sure-fire way to push the reset button and shake it all loose: Laughing!

Laughing really is good medicine, not just for the body, but for the soul. The ability to laugh is something we share with other great apes, including chimpanzees and gorillas, suggesting that it is a behavioral adaptation rooted deep in our DNA and bestowing evolutionary benefits. Laughter induces good moods and increases our capacity to learn new things, as well as helping us to build and maintain social connections.

The pleasant mental health benefits of laughing with Mike (one of the funniest people I've ever met with a wicked eye for impersonating people, famous and otherwise) last long after the last chuckle dissipates; I know for a fact that when I laugh until I almost pee my pants with my best friend, Irene, I am happy and recharged for a couple of days minimum. Surely anecdotal evidence has to count for something, but just in case my word isn't enough, along comes the Mayo Clinic, announcing that the health benefits of laughter are no joke.

They report that there are short-term benefits to tickling your funny bone: The physical act of laughing stimulates many internal organs, including your heart and lungs, enhances intake of oxygen-rich air, and increases endorphin release. A hearty laugh will also stimulate circulation and aid muscle relaxation, which both help to reduce some of the symptoms of chronic stress.

In an interesting experiment conducted in 2012, participants' pain tolerance was often increased by as much as 50% after watching a comedy video clip compared to those watching a golf how-to clip. Yes, please, I'll have some of that!

Laughing isn't just a quick-fix for what ails you. There are long-term benefits as well, not the least of which involves the release of neuropeptides that fight stress and more serious illnesses. As we found earlier, negative thoughts really do manifest chemical reactions that have serious consequences for our long-term health and well-being, and laughter is the antidote.

One organization that really gets this whole laughter thing is Gilda's Club, founded in 1989 by comedian and actor Gene Wilder after the death of his wife, comedienne Gilda Radner, from ovarian cancer. I am fortunate to be a member of the Grand Rapids, Michigan, chapter of Gilda's Club, in a big, beautiful old house whose activities are always free to me and other cancer survivors (as well as their families). The price of admission is simply that we are members of what Gilda referred to as "the elite club that no one wants to be a member of."

They have a wide variety of ongoing support groups and classes each month, including classes led by certified Laughter Yoga leaders and other classes designed to get you laughing out loud. Supporting this amazing organization locally is our local LaughFest that once a year draws headline comedy performers (including, recently, the magnificent Betty White) to Michigan for a week of pure entertainment in the middle of our brutally long, cold winter. Several of my friends surprised me with tickets to one of the shows right after my surgery, and it was just what the doctor ordered for both hubby and me.

*How to add more play and laughter to your life*

- If you live in southwest Michigan, go to the LaughFest! If not so lucky as to be nearby, seek out a comedy club.
- Watch movies and television shows that you know make you laugh.
- Hang out with a couple of kids and get goofy with them. Color in a coloring book. Wear a tiara and have a tea party. Get down on the floor and build a Lego project, or a blanket fort. Volunteer at your local children's museum.
- Buy a hula hoop. I started hula hooping with my friend Lisa the Hoop Queen right after my treatment was done, and I am here to tell you that it is impossible to hula hoop with a frown on your face. (It's a surprisingly great workout, too.)

- Join a Gilda's Club and take one of their humor-inducing and laughter-inspired classes, including Laughter Yoga.
- Even without the assistance of children, remember the lost art of play. Play like you used to years ago by immersing yourself in a creative project that reconnects you to that beautiful inner spirit that still lives and breathes deep inside.
- Go to YouTube and search for "breast cancer humor." You'll find quite a bit of it. Make a special effort to find survivor and comedienne Tig Notaro's "Hello, I Have Cancer" on iTunes. Funny. Poignant. Go see her if you ever get the chance!
- As my friend Ginjah Knuth, of FlameDancing Yoga, tells students, "And now, to perfect the advanced position of this pose, please curl the corners of your lips all the way up to your cheeks."

### The JOYFIT Project

In the midst of the final edit of this book (literally on the very last day before it was sent to print production), to my absolute delight and surprise, the universe sent me a new friend (through an old friend).

I was introduced to the amazing, energetic, highly trained, and incredibly knowledgeable Sue Ansari, a registered nurse and fellow Michigander, who not only was the first female Laughter Yoga teacher in the US, but also the person responsible for bringing Laughter Yoga to LaughFest and to Gilda's Club Grand Rapids. Additionally, she is a board certified lymphatic therapist, raw food chef, and is, herself, a breast cancer survivor.

Our synchronicity does not end there! As I wrap this up, Sue is in the midst of launching a nationwide breast cancer survivorship program, The JOYFIT Project, which incorporates everything I've talked about in *Ultimate Survivorship*.

You know, there are moments when I lose track of the deep grace and generosity of the survivorship community, times when I am so busy tending the metaphorical flowers and pulling the metaphorical weeds of this project that I forget to lay down in the grass and look up at the sky and to feel the breeze on my cheeks.

It seems that whenever that happens, I am sent an unexpected gift from the universe, and I am reminded that I am not alone on this journey. See how that works? (My gratitude continues to multiply.)

But I digress.

In a nutshell, Sue describes The JOYFIT Project as "an innovative new whole body wellness program that combines the best of holistic mind, body, and spirit modalities to educate, enlighten, and encourage breast cancer survivors on how to live a JoyFULL life, during and after a cancer diagnosis."

## Components of The JOYFIT Project

- Laughter Yoga to increase lymphatic flow, decrease stress, and elevate mood.
- Specific movements that are custom-designed to open lymphatic pathways, while reducing existing lymphedema and reducing the risk of developing it.
- Plant-based, unprocessed whole food recipes designed to be not only easy, tasty, and delicious for the entire family, but specifically designed to reduce the risk of cancer recurrence.
- Meditation techniques to improve emotional and physical well being.
- The bonds of a female community support group to empower, encourage, and enable survivors to eat, exercise, and think their way into the healthiest, happiest versions of themselves.

## THE BOTTOM LINE

That's right, please remember to smile as often as you can. Make time each and every day to laugh and to play. It isn't just our genetic birthright—it's one of the ways we can make an intentional decision as to how to handle this whole breast cancer situation, which tends to be a serious business when left to its own devices.

Remembering to connect with our playful, childlike, and humorous natures will take us to a higher place, one where we can view our sometimes chaotic worlds from a different perspective, one that is more relaxed, positive, joyful, and emotionally balanced.

And finally, seek out a JOYFIT class near you, as Sue Ansari expands across the country. You will undoubtedly be hearing more about The JOYFIT Project (including web links) on the companion website to *Ultimate Survivorship*, as we both strive to follow our life's work, educating and supporting breast cancer survivors across the country.

# 38. VISUALIZE WHAT YOU NEED MOST

Radiation was a seven-week-and-33-dose-long treatment phase for me and was, without a doubt, the most dehumanizing experience of my personal lifetime. It was the only time in my entire life that I briefly stopped writing. I later described how I felt about radiation treatments. It was like this.

*Radiation memories*

Imagine that you have been working on a beautiful, sunny Saturday morning to spring-clean your house from top to bottom. The music is playing full blast and you are singing all the songs loud and happy because it's Aretha and you always clean loud and happy with Aretha. First you wash all of the windows, including the sliding door to the deck. In and out that door you go all morning, stopping to take breaks in the sun before resuming.

The afternoon cools and you slide the door shut, heading upstairs for the next big push. Dangit! You left the mop on the deck and scoot down there to get it, still singing. You spy the bucket on the deck and rush toward it, running *smacksmacksmacksmacksmack* into the door, completely forgetting that you had shut it.

That's what it was like for me, except the happy cleaning frenzy meant "healing after surgery," and the happy singing meant "the love of my friends and how quickly I am healing and how incredible and whole I feel," and the sliding door meant "radiation treatments," and the *smacksmacksmack* thing meant "well, girlie, we're so glad you think you have this whole breast cancer situation all dealt with, but in case you forgot while you were skipping down the street and meditating and being all filled with the love of your friends and family and smiling and feeling cured, by the way, *you might fucking still have cancer*, so now we're gonna shoot you with whatever the product of a linear accelerator is every day for the next couple of months in the hopes that we kill a couple more stray cancer cells, that's how much you need to want to not die, and that's how serious this really is, just in case you forgot, so you just lay yourself down on this here lead table and close your eyes and we'll play you some music and shut you in a lead bunker behind this enormously thick lead door, and please excuse us while we jog to the other side of that enormous lead door, in fact as far and as fast away as we can manage before we flip the little switch."

Kinda like that, but slightly more terrifying. (And I do apologize somewhat for my vulgarity, but that is the truth, and there is no prettier way to express it. There just isn't.)

I had breezed through Blue Dot Day, where I got the tiny (and permanent) tattoos used to line me up on the machine, and I had breezed right through simulation and practice days, so when Mike asked if I needed him to come along again the first day, I said, "Nah, I'm good." Then the *smack* thing happened, and I sat in the parking lot after the first dose and put my head down on the steering wheel and cried, remembering that I really did have cancer.

So he went with me for a while after that, until I calmed myself down and got really good at visualizations, affirmations, and self-talk.


*Visualizations got me through*


The actual radiation only takes a few seconds, and then the accelerator hums to another position and starts up again. After that first time, I prepared myself with a few cleansing breaths and waited for a visualization to appear. My favorite at one low point was "Laser Cats," modeled after a Saturday Night Live sketch of the same name, which helped me to smile, which gave me courage. Sound effect: Pew. Pew-pew. Pew-pew-pew!

When they turned it on, the Varian with which they radiated me sounded like a hive of bees. Sometimes I saw them swarming into my breast on a fat cloud of white light and feeding on cancer cells like nectar. Some days I pictured myself lying on a beach, the sun baking my chest and evaporating the stray cells. I had quite a few different visualizations, and I didn't make them up as much as wait for them to appear.

Because the radiation treatments were so quick, I spent more time with visualizations at home than there. I do love them and still use them whenever I want a free mini-vacation at a moments' notice.

My treatment visualizations progressed from pre-surgery healing white lights and butterflies, to the crazy laser cats, bees, and beaches, and finally, at the very end, pure electrical energy that vaporized what was left of the errant cells and gave me just enough spunk to get in the car and drive home.

Every day a new healing fantasy made its way into my thoughts. I am grateful for a healthy imagination, but if you could use a boost in that regard, pick up the lyrical and delightful *Joy is a Plum-Colored Acrobat* by Wendy Burton. She sets up quite a variety of visualizations to use during different phases of treatment. I think her goal is for you to try a few on for size and use them to spark adaptations and variations that really speak to you on a deeply personal level.

Several friends (and friends of friends) have found Dr. Neil Neimark's *Less Stress Surgery* to be tremendously helpful. Relying on the most recent research in the area of behavioral anesthesiology, Dr. Neimark's guided imagery relaxation may help speed your recovery, minimize post-operative pain, and decrease anxiety in general. Another practitioner of guided imagery that comes highly recommended is Belleruth Naparstek, who has a plethora of topics to choose from, including visualizations to help fight cancer, minimize anxiety, promote successful surgery, and ease pain.

*Not all visualizations are helpful*

Worry is one example of negative visualization that may seize control of your brain in ways that aren't productive to your goals and desires. For this reason, practicing positive visualizations to replace them will help.

One such technique is a classic called simply The Pink Bubble. Try it for yourself if you wish: Sitting or lying down comfortably, close your eyes and establish a calm, deep rhythm of breathing. Notice the negative or worrying thought that has been showing up to cause distress. Place it into a short sentence. Now, picture the actual words that make up this sentence, and gently enclose the words in a pink bubble. Allow the words, and the soft pink bubble, to disappear into the universe, along with your negative thought.

## THE BOTTOM LINE

We have substantial power to change the direction of our thought process, and the physical processes that ultimately follow, by visualizing the very things that we need most, whether it is healing, calm, peace, or a desired outcome.

Can we create the outcome we so desperately wish to happen? Probably not, but it sure is worth a go, and in the meanwhile gives us a sense of strength and participation in an often dehumanizing treatment process.

## 39. SPEAK TO (AND OF) YOURSELF AS THOUGH YOU ARE A DEAR FRIEND

Positive self-talk, also referred to as self-affirmation, can be an effective tool for coping with the ongoing emotional complications of treatment and survivorship, including anxiety, stress, depression, and PTSD, which, left unattended to simmer and brew, can double in on themselves to multiply and flourish. Lymphedema, fertility issues, fatigue, fear of recurrence, sex problems, and negative body image all do their parts to give us the push our minds need to descend into even more dark and scary territory.

Positive self-talk statements are realistic (generally present-tense) sentences you intentionally construct about yourself or a situation, spoken in the first person. This technique has been shown to have a considerable impact on our ability to cope with breast cancer treatment and the physical and emotional aftermath.

It seems that sometimes we just need to practice the fine art of noticing things that aren't easy to notice when we are busy noticing the really big things that are right in front of our faces. It's all there if we pay attention.

*Don't get me wrong:*
*I'm willing to experience negative emotions*

And, by the way, using this technique does not mean that you are plugging your ears, shutting your eyes, and humming "happy birthday to me" over and over in a ridiculous attempt to pretend that there's nothing going on, nothing upsetting or frightening you, or pretending that everything is just fine, thank you very much, when that is clearly not true.

This is not, I repeat *not*, an avoidance technique, but rather a way of ap-

173

proaching the difficulties you are facing in a calmer, more proactive, and most decidedly more productive way.

What do you do if you tend to think the worst, or are a full-fledged pessimist? Just know that if you do the mental work to identify your negative thinking patterns and thoughts, you have the power to make actual changes to the way your mind processes information.

You are not required to be a mere recipient of whatever random thoughts appear in your mind. You have the power to be not only an editor but the actual creator of your own reality, and the very first step in this process is to begin to identify the negative self-talk that you are allowing. Psychologists identify a few different types of negative thinking patterns.

### Filtering

Filtering is one of the most common negative thinking patterns we easily find ourselves engaged in, for humans in general, but especially for people in crisis mode. We start to only notice the bad things, the things that are hurting us or making us fearful and may cause us to forget (filter out) that there are still wonderful things happening in our lives and in the world. How easy it is to notice only the bad when we're going through the sadness, discomfort, pain, and indignities of treatment!

### All-or-nothing

All-or-nothing thinking is a way of looking at the world in a black-or-white, good-or-bad, win-or-lose kind of a way, forgetting that there are quite a few shades of gray (Actually, I heard there were 50. Just sayin'.)

### Catastrophizing

Catastrophizing is just that: You pretty much begin to expect the worst to always be heading your way. Woe is me!

### Overgeneralization

Overgeneralization is when we come to an overarching conclusion on a particular subject based on scant evidence: I'm late, everyone is staring at me, and the doctor hates me!

*Emotional reasoning*

Emotional reasoning is when we allow ourselves to be so overwhelmed by our feelings that we begin to mistake them for facts. When you are *feeling* hopeless, you interpret that to mean that things *are* hopeless.

*Should statements*

Should statements set up unrealistic expectations for you, your family, your doctors, and the world at large that don't allow for flexibility, reality, or set-backs. Go easy on yourself, girl.

*And others: we are so very creative*

And there are others. We like to take responsibility for things that are clearly not our fault (like our cancer). We love to read other people's minds and to make negative assumptions about what they are thinking. We have the ability to predict the future. We have a tendency to exaggerate the importance of negative information, or conversely, we trivialize the importance of something that is really huge. We also like to assign blame, and sometimes, to put labels on ourselves and others.

Holy smokes, girls! The things that we do to ourselves, the additional weight that we put on our own shoulders, is astounding.

The good news in all of this is that, with practice, we can replace these negative and distorted patterns of thinking, patterns that cause us harm, with new and positive patterns that become our allies, because we have the absolute power to change, "I can't do this," into, "How can I make it happen?"

*Negative self-talk*

To follow are a few examples of negative self-talk statements that are by their very nature limiting and defeating, followed shortly by some replacement phrases. One way to assess what you are thinking is to ask yourself, "If I were my own best friend, would I say this to myself?" Would you say any of these things to someone you genuinely cared about?

"This is too hard and too complicated."

"I don't understand anything the doctor is saying."

"There is no way in the whole wide world I can do this."

"I'm too stupid, (scared, lazy, broke) to go through this."

"I'm never going to be myself ever again."

"I've done it another way too long to change."

"I shouldn't be such a sissy/so scared/so fearful."

"Everyone else handles things better than I do."

"I know this surgery is going to be a disaster!"

### Stewart Smiley

There are some that deny the power of affirmations, or tell me that they are silly or ridiculous, picturing the character Stewart Smiley on the old SNL skit: "I'm good enough, I'm smart enough, and doggone it, people like me!" (I always loved Stewart and wanted to give him a hug.) It seems to me that this criticism would more reasonably be directed toward affirmations that aren't honest or those that are just wishes.

For example, if the negative thought, "I'm scared," is simply turned on its head and becomes the supposed affirmation, "I'm not scared," repeating over and over to yourself that you aren't scared, when, in fact, you are scared out of your ever-loving mind, not only doesn't make you feel less scared, but in all probability might scare you even more!

So my thought is that when you are working on positive self-talk statements, please don't use statements of denial that will serve to hurt you even more in the long run. I've found that, oftentimes, the simple act of acknowledging my negative emotions gives me the power to move beyond them. Don't be afraid to be fully afraid.

### Deep within

Further, while I am not in the least sense of the word religious, I think of affirmations as prayers to myself that, though from moment to moment experiencing some of the most frightening thoughts a person can have, allow me to access the strength and courage that I know is inside me.

My very best affirmations resonate with my own truth, my own power, and come from a place deep within, a place where I am speaking to myself as a friend would. How would you move differently through your day if the negative thoughts expressed earlier were intentionally re-phrased?

*Positive self-talk*

"Yes, this is hard and this is complicated, but I can ask for help and there are many willing to give me help. I can write questions down, and I can ask all the questions I need to, until I understand as best I can."

"The doctor is using words that I don't understand. I can ask him to explain in more detail."

"I am feeling overwhelmed because there is so much to figure out. I don't have to do everything today, and I can take this one step at a time."

"I am doing the very best that I can to make my way through this experience with grace and courage."

"No matter the outcome, I can never be anyone but myself. I welcome the deepening of my spirit through this process."

"I know I have the power to create dramatic change for the better in my life. I am the creator of my future. I hold my own destiny."

"Of course I am scared! This is a scary thing I am dealing with. But I am also working to access all of the wisdom, courage and strength I know is inside me."

"I am coping with this in the best way that I can, using the information that I have, and working to make positive changes for my future."

"I am nervous about my surgery. I am confident I chose the right doctor for this surgery. She knows what she is doing and has done this many times."

*Give yourself unconditional love*

You are about to embark on a life-altering series of changes that will transform your body and reverberate through your life in many ways. The changes that are being discussed are not by way of blaming you, or shaming you for what you have done, or not done, or neglected to do, or forgot to do, or were too busy to do, to find yourself in this predicament.

This is not about knocking yourself around for those extra pounds or about disliking the beautiful woman you see in the mirror, because yup, you are a beautiful woman, even with your clothes in a heap on the floor and the lights turned all the way up.

And this isn't about being more courageous than the next woman. Many souls who have fought hard and done everything they possibly could have lost the fight anyway. This isn't about comparing yourself to me (or me comparing myself to another) and coming up short in the comparison. You are exactly where you need to be. You are exactly who you need to be, in this time, and for this moment.

This is a different trip, a trip that begins with genuine love and deep compassion for the woman you are right now, in this place in your life, with all of your amazing imperfections and quirks and characteristics that make you so perfectly you and no one else on this big blue marble hurtling relentlessly through space.

We are not striving for perfection but, much more simply, seeking to find a healthy and adaptive response to one of the most challenging experiences of our lifetimes. It's a process, and you'll do the best that you can, whatever that is.

## THE BOTTOM LINE

I am sometimes scared for what the future might hold, and that's okay, because cancer can be a scary thing. I honor this fear and give it a place in my heart. And then I move forward to learn new ways to take care of myself, find new information that gives my life more depth and meaning.

I give myself the compassion and respect I give those around me, and I strive to compare myself to no one but me. I find productive ways to replace fear with knowledge. I empower myself to move beyond my fear, returning from time to time to experience it again in all of its richness and intensity and realness.

I refuse to fall into a never-ending chasm of despair or hopelessness. Even if I knew with certainty that the situation was dire, I swear I would strive to fill each of my days, each of my hours and minutes, with as much love and passion for what remained as I could scrape together.

# 40. SEEK OUT A MINDFULNESS-BASED STRESS REDUCTION CLASS

It seems that there are just about as many variations on the practice of meditation as there are people practicing it: Autogenic training, Ayurveda, Brahma Kumaris, Raja yoga, breathing awareness, Chi Kung, guided imagery and meditation, loving-kindness, mantra, Omkar, relaxation response, sitting, standing, and walking meditations, that Trademarked Meditation, Vairochana posture, vipassana, zazen and Zen, to name just a few that I ran across as I researched this topic.

The art of meditation has been practiced for thousands of years on all continents, most particularly emanating from Eastern philosophical traditions. In contemporary times, and most particularly in Western traditions, meditation is usually practiced outside of any religious context. This is the practice discussed here, although there is no reason you couldn't incorporate an element of your particular faith if it meant something to you.

### Monkey-mind

Humans embody a nature that has for centuries been referred to as monkey-mind. Seemingly random thoughts fight for a place in the front of our brains, the streaming consciousness of thoughts piled upon thoughts that fill our days from the moment we wake up until the moment we hit the pillow, and in times of crisis such as this, very often noisily try to elbow their way into the time we should be using to sleep, as well.

The monkeys in our minds pull our thoughts this way and that, incessantly re-hashing the past and worrying about the tomorrow: Plotting, planning, scheming for the future, always busy commenting and judging even the tiniest minutiae of our experience.

This constant and uncontrolled monkey-mind chatter is the primary thing that prevents us from enjoying the only moment that truly exists: This one. The past has fled, riding a wave of fluidly changing memory. The future seductively beckons us to race ahead, away from what we have sitting right in front of us this very second. Mindfulness practice is a simple and effective approach to meditation in which your attention is deliberately focused on a physical sensation in the present, such as your breath.

When thoughts intrude into our mindfulness practice (as they will, because you are a human being), you will simply notice them, without judgment, and return to the focus. In this way, you practice drawing yourself away from thoughts of other moments, past or present, in order to more deeply and fully experience what we have right now. The goal is a simple one: To seek moment to moment nonjudgmental awareness.

## Jon Kabat-Zinn's MBSR

One program that was created around this goal is Mindfulness-Based Stress Reduction (MBSR), developed by Jon Kabat-Zinn and colleagues at the University of Massachusetts in the late 70's and 80's, a program that has now expanded worldwide. MBSR is firmly rooted in the contemplative arts, in which an individual actively cultivates conscious awareness.

Within the basic framework developed by Zinn, the personal qualities of nonjudgment, acceptance, and patience are practiced and enhanced in a meditation that typically focuses on the breath, which leads to a state not only of relaxation but of healthy detachment from the emotional stress of living with an essentially chronic condition such as breast cancer.

The body of scientific evidence has grown significantly through the years, pointing to MBSR's statistically relevant fourfold result: A reduction in stress, perceived improvement of quality of life, reaching a deeper sense of meaning and purpose in life, and experiencing a greater sense of perceived wellness.

When I ran across this technique, I was fully immersed in survivorship research. As I reviewed programs online and learned more about it, I realized that MBSR was another meaningful way to actively participate in my medical treatment.

Early on, I decided to take personal accountability for every choice I made, looking to myself for learning, growing, healing and transforming my life as a breast cancer survivor. In my opinion, this program might very well be the best first step you can take in regard to such goals. All else will flow nicely from this beginning: Mindful eating, exercising, love, relationships . . . and mindful ultimate survivorship!

*It works*

In an article published in the April 20, 2012, *Journal of Clinical Oncology*, Hoffman *et al* reported the findings of a randomized and controlled study of 229 women in treatment for stage 0 to III breast cancer who underwent MBSR training. The researchers found statistically significant improvement in outcome for total mood disturbance (including anxiety and depression), anger, lack of vigor, fatigue, and confusion, as well as improvement in indicators of physical, social, emotional, and functional well-being.

They concluded that MBSR improved mood, breast- and endocrine-related quality of life and well-being and that the effects persisted after the training was completed. Numerous studies have repeated these results.

Depression is one of the best-studied behavioral side-effects of breast cancer treatment. Up to half of all women treated have reported it as a problem in their lives to one degree or another, even if minor. Most studies, however, find that roughly 20-30% of women actively in treatment experience elevated depressive symptoms, with 9% of ambulatory breast cancer patients experiencing a true clinical depression (defined as lasting at least two weeks and causing significant impairment in social functioning).

Depression can play a huge role in quality of life and can be associated with less concern for following medical treatment requirements. There is also some evidence of increased mortality in depressed cancer patients.

MBSR intervention has been found to be effective in reducing depressive symptoms in at least two ways: By buffering the way you can focus on the negative aspects of yourself and what's going on in your life, and by reducing the frequency of purely emotional responses to life situations.

*So what does the MBSR program look like?*

The training that I participated in at the local Gilda's Club is pretty typical. It included eight weeks of classes as well as a one day silent retreat toward the end. Each class is roughly two and a half hours long (once a week at the same time) and includes three basic learning components.

There is usually an orientation session before the class begins, during which the program is outlined and you can ask questions. You'll also have to agree to do the homework, which consists of daily practice of one or more of the techniques and journaling about your experiences.

In each class, participants sit in a circle, wearing comfortable clothing, and are given instruction on one of the meditation techniques, which might include one of the sitting meditations (sitting with breath, sitting with breath and the body, sitting with sound, sitting with thoughts and feelings, and sitting with choiceless awareness, for example) or the body scan technique. This is followed by a mindful movement such as yoga, qigong, or walking meditation.

Participants in MBSR class will learn a great deal through lectures and discussions, including how habitual knee-jerk reactions create anxiety, depression, and illness, as well as how to work to change those responses to the stress in their lives. There is typically time in each class for participants to share their experiences as they practice these new stress-reduction techniques and to ask questions.

As I mentioned, the MBSR training that I attended was through the local Gilda's Club, truly one of the most beautiful places in existence for people with cancer and their loved ones. Membership and all classes and activities, and by this I mean everything you ever do at Gilda's Club, is free for you and your caregiver. Every meal shared, each class participated in, every book borrowed, is free.

The price of admission is simply that you are a cancer survivor or a caregiver. I truly could not love the people that make this possible any more than I do. It is a grace-filled house, and I am grateful that it exists.

## THE BOTTOM LINE

My best advice is to ask the social worker at your doctor's office for help finding free classes you can sign up for either at Gilda's Club (if you are fortunate enough to have one nearby) or through other local organizations, hospitals, or clinics. Many mindfulness practices may also have scholarships for cancer patients.

If you can't find a free class, I am telling you straight up that this is worth every nickel, and then a thousand more, if you end up having to pay for the class out-of-pocket. I also found a huge number of online MBSR training programs. Look for one that has been around for awhile (and, therefore, is more likely to have the bugs worked out for the online piece of it) and that the instructor has been trained in MBSR.

If you are unable to take the class (and I truly hope that isn't the case), there are inexpensive and high-quality books and videos widely available that you can use in your mindfulness study and practice on your own.

# 41. SCHEDULE A MASSAGE
## (OR THREE)

We are well aware that stress, anxiety, and depression can result in a decrease in natural killer cells, which has been linked to increased tumor development, and we've discussed the links between stress, inflammation, and cancer growth in just about every topic covered in this book. The healing arts, including the energy arts, have much to offer us, not just during treatment and recovery, but in our happily-ever-after, as well.

Massage therapy in particular offers tremendous evidence-based physical and emotional benefits to breast cancer survivors. And, seriously, I look for just about any excuse in the world to book a massage.

A small but important preliminary study published in 2010 by a division of the National Institutes of Health found that volunteers who received just one 45-minute Swedish massage experienced significant decreases in levels of the stress hormone cortisol, as well as the hormonal precursors to cortisol. The volunteers also increased lymphocyte production, which are the white blood cells of the immune system.

In an earlier study, women diagnosed with breast cancer who received massage therapy (three 30-minute sessions a week) for five weeks reported less depressed mood, anxiety, and pain at the end of the study. Dopamine (happy hormones), natural killer cells, and lymphocytes also increased. These findings are backed up by a significant amount of research on the health benefits of therapeutic massage.

Massage therapy should be administered by a licensed massage therapist experienced in dealing with the physical issues that come with breast cancer treatment. This is especially important if you are currently experiencing any physical symptoms, including lymphedema, radiation burn, mastectomy pain, or are presently in chemotherapy. During chemo, blood count for platelets and/or lymphocytes often drop below normal levels, and it's important that your therapist be experienced in working with our particular set of side effects before proceeding.

You can find a professional, nationally-certified massage therapist through the National Certification Board for Therapeutic Massage and Bodywork or the American Massage Therapy Association. I would suggest that you start with recommendations from your medical team, physical therapist, nurse navigator, or another survivor that has had a positive experience with a local therapist.

### *How to choose a massage therapist*

My dear friend Beth, a massage therapist in New Hampshire, gave me valuable advice on how to go about choosing a massage therapist.

"Bottom line, don't just pick somebody off the website and trust it. Call. Ask questions: How long have you been a massage therapist? Where did you learn to work with people who have cancer? How long have you been working with people who have cancer? What would I need to do to make sure our work is safe for me? The answers you get to this last one are particularly revealing—you don't want a blithe panacea.

"You also want them to ask *you* questions about your treatment and your physical condition. You want them to describe how they would work with you and how they would interact with your medical team. You want them to sound like they know what they are doing and are not scared of the job. And you want them to sound like someone you feel comfortable with on a personality basis."

I know she is a therapist willing to have these conversations with potential clients with special needs or concerns. It's important to her that the client-therapist match is a good one, and in my opinion, a therapist who isn't willing to take a few minutes to speak with you, or is offended by straightforward questions about qualifications and experience, gets scratched right off the list. The therapist should also have a new client intake form to learn about any medications or conditions that are contraindications or areas of special concern.

### THE BOTTOM LINE

This is a not just a matter of pampering yourself (body and soul). I consider massage an essential part of my health maintenance program. Find a massage professional who has experience working with breast cancer survivors.

# 42. EXPLORE GENTLE
# MINDFULNESS-BASED EXERCISE

There is a fair amount of research suggesting that mindfulness-based exercise, including yoga, qigong, and tai chi, offers substantial benefit to cancer patients, not just for relieving side effects of treatment, but for improvement of physical function and an increased quality of life.

## *Yoga*

Yoga is a combination of physical postures and poses we are all familiar with as well as elements of breathing techniques and meditation derived from the ancient Hindu religious practice of Yoga with a capital Y. The non-religious practice of yoga with a lower case y has been modified throughout the years and adapted for use in Western cultures to promote physical and mental control and well-being. (If you are a religious or spiritual person, these beliefs can become a component of your yoga practice.)

Yoga provided significant improvements in breast cancer survivors' fatigue in one 12-week study. Other trials report significantly better overall perception of health as well as physical and psychological functioning in women going through radiation treatments for stages 0 to II breast cancer. Also reported were less fatigue and insomnia, higher quality of life, social, and emotional well-being and spirituality after chemotherapy treatment, less nausea, and a smaller decrease in natural killer cells between diagnosis and the end of chemo.

A review published in the December 2012 journal *Supportive Care in Cancer* concluded that there is "moderate to good evidence" that yoga may be a useful practice for women recovering from breast cancer treatments.

## *Qigong*

My first working experience with qigong (chee-gong) was when my friend Debby sent me a beautiful, pampering care package filled to the brim with healing gifts including amazing teas, snacks, lotions, and potions . . . so many perfectly appropriate gifts, I was slightly overwhelmed.

One of the gifts was a beginning qigong DVD. I opened it up right away and started practicing the gentle, flowing, healing movements. The practice of qigong includes slow body movements and meditation, often with mental imagery, and sometimes not. I found in my research that there are literally hundreds of different types of qigong, also called chi gung.

Qigong incorporates specific techniques that are particularly effective for specific diseases, including cancer. For example, there are methods for easing the effects of radiation and chemotherapy. One method used for this is called dragon and tiger medical qigong, sometimes called "meridian-line qigong" because it helps by balancing the chi flow that some believe runs through energy channels of your body. (And if nothing else, is calming and relaxing.)

Most of the research on qigong has been done on healthy adults. One small study in particular concluded that regular qigong practice lowered stress hormone levels along with cytokine-secreting blood cells, which we are well aware by now, means that there was a reduction in stress levels in the volunteers.

Another study, on patients with chronic pain issues, showed that qigong may be useful as a complementary strategy for managing stress in cancer patients; the training was associated with short-term pain reduction and long-term anxiety reduction. Additional research strongly suggests that medical qigong benefits cognitive function, quality of life, and the inflammation process, as well as providing fatigue and mood improvements.

## *Tai chi and tai chi chuan*

Tai chi (tie-gee), also referred to as tai chi chuan, is another gentle and mindful practice that many have confused with qigong. (Sigh. This includes me. Frankly, I couldn't tell the difference if my life depended on it at this point.) Discussion abounds on the topic, and if you are really interested you can look for more information than I am planning to give you on these pages.

Tai chi chuan is a mindful exercise practice that has positive effects on aerobic capacity, strength, and quality of life among cancer survivors. One pilot study assessed the effects of a 12-week tai chi chuan class and found stable insulin levels in the test group (compared to a non-exercising group), concluding further that positive changes in cytokine levels could be important for maintaining lean body mass in breast cancer survivors.

Two well-designed studies of tai chi chuan in breast cancer survivors reported significant differences in psychological and physiological symptoms when compared to a group that only had therapeutic support. Tai chi practice resulted in improved aerobic capacity, strength, flexibility, body composition, self-esteem, quality of life, and immune function among breast cancer patients in a whole slew of studies.

## THE BOTTOM LINE

Finding the time to incorporate gentle and mindful exercise into our daily routines will offer benefits galore as we move into the survivorship years. Whether a class or on DVD, explore the healing arts from this gentle new perspective.

# 43. ON MOTIVATION

It would seem logical that every single woman diagnosed with breast cancer (or any disease that has connections to lifestyle, for that matter) would be automatically and naturally compelled to make deep and wide changes in the way she goes about her life's business.

And yet, it isn't so. In a way, I am mystified by this reaction, but in a way, not. Human beings have that part of the brain that actively resists change, a part that fights with all its formidable weaponry for the status quo, even when the status quo is causing harm.

Our ego constantly reminds us that change is hard, that other people will think we're weird, that it doesn't matter, anyway, that we like things just exactly the way they are, that we're going to die anyway someday, that life just isn't worth living without the foods that we know and love and that have given us comfort and sustenance all these years, that our knees hurt too much to walk every day, that we are too old to make changes.

And so, to begin this journey with me will be a period of work and transition. (Which is a reminder of my childbirth experience, hard work indeed, most specifically the transition phase, just moments before each of the girls was born, when I looked at the father of my children and advised him, with every fiber of my being, that he would never touch me again as long as I drew breath. Both times. Ah, life.)

It is, however, work that will pay great dividends. Here are some thoughts on how to dig deep and find the motivation to make important life changes.

*Make decisions and describe the result*

The very first step is to make an actual, concrete decision to enact the changes that you wish to make. Write down short sentences filled with verbs. Give yourself deadlines and time frames. A sentence that reflects a vague decision along the lines of, "I plan to eat healthier," becomes, "I will transition to a 100% whole foods, plant-based diet within the next twelve months." "I will become fit," turns into, "I will exercise for three to five hours a week effective immediately," and, "I need to lose weight," into, "I will lose ten pounds in the next six months."

### *Learn how to eat an elephant*

I am fortunate to have volunteered with Mediation Services in Holland, Michigan, since 2006. One of my peacemaking partners, Pat, often tells stories that illustrate points he wishes to make in mediation sessions, and several of his favorites involve elephants. Once we have completed the task of creating an agenda for the session, the participants almost invariably look at the whiteboard filled with difficult topics for discussion, glance across the table at the people sitting there, people with whom they've been at war for months (or even years) and are frequently overwhelmed with the seemingly insurmountable issues on the table.

We see quite a few deer-in-the headlights expressions right about this time, which prompts Pat to ask: "Do you guys know how to eat an elephant?" Of course, we are met with head-shakes in the negative, which allows him to respond, "One bite at a time."

Whatever it is you want to do, once you have decided the "what" of it, break it down into smaller steps. A goal that seeks transition to a whole foods, plant-based diet in twelve months is broken down into smaller goals with smaller incremental time frames. Is there an element of education involved in your decision? Make that one of the steps, and decide how you're going to go about that.

### *Hang out with cheerleaders*

I can practically guarantee that you are going to be met with resistance by friends and family members who are not themselves committed to the changes you wish to make. You are going to be challenged and tested and questioned.

Avoid saboteurs with every fiber of your being; positive changes can be threatening to others. Make the whole darn thing easier by surrounding yourself with cheerleaders who think you're awesome and who admire you for wanting to take the trajectory of your life into your own hands.

If that isn't your spouse, or close girlfriend, or family, make sure that you somehow find yourself a buddy (or a whole group of buddies) who share your goals and dreams. When I signed up for a half marathon with my daughter Rachel, I immediately began to train with a running club whose members ran together on a regular basis. It held me accountable and offered a system of support that got me through to race day. (I try to pick something impossible to do each year in honor of being alive. Running a real half marathon with Rachel was one of the first impossible things I decided to do once I was recovered.)

### *Say it out loud*

Tell people what you are doing. Talk about it in positive ways. "I am quitting smoking." "I am excited to be changing my eating habits for the better." (And then recruit their support.)

### *Identify and eliminate limiting beliefs*

Do not allow yourself to be held back by limiting beliefs that might be knocking around in your head. Is age 50 too old to start making dramatic changes in your life? I think not. Find examples of people who overcame the limitations you think belong to you, and know that you can do it, too.

For pure inspiration, look up a YouTube video, *Arthur's Transformation*, made by Arthur Boorman, an obese 47-year-old disabled Gulf War paratrooper who was told that he would never walk unassisted again.

The video documents his journey from 100% disability to health, wellness, and vitality. As Arthur advises, "Never underestimate what you can accomplish when you believe in yourself." Whenever I think that I have bit off more than I can chew in any area of my life, I turn to Arthur's video for a reminder of what is truly possible. Own your life!

### *Acknowledge successes*

When you complete one of the steps outlined in your plan, remember to acknowledge what you have done and then give yourself a reward.

### *Plan menus*

I find that one of the most important steps I take as I continue this journey involves preparation, the act of looking ahead so that stumbling blocks don't blindside me. For example, I plan most of my meals in advance and spend blocks of time preparing more than one meal. I'm not quite as organized as those remarkable people who plan weeks or even months in advance, but I do try to plan for a week at a time.

Mostly, my menu planning revolves around the produce picked up on my most recent marketing foray followed by rummaging through the pantry and freezer to see what is available and looks good there, as well. I always have a cookbook on the nightstand, and give Mike the task of finding recipes that look good to him from time to time.

### *Plan food for work and for on the road*

I work long hours on weekends, and unhealthy, unacceptable food is everywhere in my workplace. It is absolutely my biggest struggle and most common place where I fall right down on my big bottom. A girlfriend gave me the idea of a rolling cooler filled with everything I might need for the long shift ahead. I haven't done that yet, as I have access to a kitchen and full-sized refrigerator at work, but I like that idea quite a bit and thought I'd pass it along to you.

On the weekends that I don't take the time to plan everything I will eat for the whole 12 hours, I find myself in deep dookie, so I make every effort not to get caught unprepared. Try to have something nutritious to eat nearby as often as you can.

### *Plan responses*

People will not understand what you are doing, they will want to tell you that you are going overboard, they will give you lectures on "moderation," and they will intentionally attempt to sabotage your efforts to make life changes. One of the best ways to counteract verbal nonsense of this nature is by having responses all loaded and ready to go for various situations that are bound to come up.

I always make sure that responses are, first of all, reminders to myself of what I am setting out to accomplish, and further, are non-judgmental. Some of the most common things I hear are along the lines of, "Just one bite won't kill you," and, "It's a celebration, go ahead and enjoy it," or, "There's only a little mayo in it, you should be fine," to which I often respond with a genuine, "Thank you so much for the offer, it looks absolutely delicious/scrumptious/divine, but I eat a whole foods, plant-based diet that doesn't include (fill in the blank: oatmeal cookies/dairy mayo/chocolate cake/ice cream/porterhouse steak), and it's important to me that I stick by my plan." I don't go into detail unless I am asked and the person sincerely wants to know.

*Schedule your priorities*

The best way to get into a new habit of including an activity in your life is by setting a schedule for it. I do carry a day planner at all times, into which I write *in ink* the activities that I need to accomplish each week, including work, medical appointments, exercise, meditation, meal planning and preparation, as well as time with my family and volunteer work.

It's amazing how much simpler it is to decline someone's kind offer to do something else when the week has already been prioritized. Of course, that's not to say that the schedule isn't up for revision. I enjoy spontaneous shenanigans and cherish every moment I spend with the people I love. Scheduled time can be rearranged as long as you are not giving up on your goals and personal priorities on a regular basis.


*Practice saying no*

You can do it. Go ahead, say it out loud: "I'm sorry, I can't. That just doesn't work for me. No thank you. No. Uh-uh. Nope."


*Keep a log*

Many women find it helpful to keep a log as they make major dietary and lifestyle changes. This will hold you accountable *to* yourself for goals you have set *for* yourself. For example, a large observational study at Kaiser Permanente found that participants who wrote down what they ate were substantially more successful in meeting their goals.

"The more food records people kept, the more weight they lost," says Jack Hollis, PhD, one of the researchers and lead author of the study, published in the August 2006 issue of the *American Journal of Preventative Medicine*. "Those who kept daily food records lost twice as much as those who kept no records at all." The simple act of writing it down was the key.

Logging doesn't have to just apply to food, but also would be a useful tool for keeping track of other important things we want to make sure to make a daily priority such as exercise, nutrients, or specific self-care goals.


*Make a vision board*

Others have found a vision board useful in reaching for their dreams. Glue pictures, motivational and inspirational quotes, headlines, and artwork on a big poster for a daily reminder of what you wish to achieve.

*Don't judge others . . . or yourself*

Remember that everyone is on their own path. We know what we know and not a whit more; we make choices based on that information, which is woven in with life experiences, what we were taught as children, and where our lives have taken us.

## THE BOTTOM LINE

The decisions you have made and the life that you wish to live may well be difficult to accomplish. There will be people who will intentionally (or not) wish for you to fail, and there will be stumbling blocks along the way. Make a plan and stick to it, finding motivation from positive people in your life and using techniques that have been proven successful. Begin right now with something simple.

Make one decision, and go with it. Today. This very second. Seriously, just do it. You may wish to begin with low-hanging fruit, so to speak, and work your way up, if that's the way you need to do it. Then get the plan formulated, and start putting one foot in front of the other.

# 44. TAKE ONE STEP

These lovely and exceptionally durable bodies we toddle around in all day long, while sometimes clumsily evolved (I'm specifically visualizing the childbirth experience here), are at the same time elegantly made—not unlike the universe from which we all spring and to which we will eventually return—with the incredible ability to restore stasis, health, and well-being.

Each day I find myself astounded at the synergistic construction of the universe and everything in it, including us. From the tiniest microbes that inhabit our bodies and without which we cannot survive, to the immense and vibrating dance of the universe itself: We are part of a system of vibrant, humming life.

And so, in this, my last essay shot straight from my heart to yours, I want to talk about harnessing the power of synergy. Because this whole thing isn't just about eating a pile of veggies and fruits (although that's wildly important). It isn't about starting to exercise. (Also important.) Or throwing mushrooms on your pizza, or drinking green tea, or (insert list of everything I have talked about as important considerations for breast cancer survivors).

It's about all of it, all of it as a whole, how it all fits together and works to allow maximum health and well being.

In the course of researching the new paradigm by which to choose the most beneficial approach to life after diagnosis, I eventually realized that I needed to re-engage my entire life in a proactive, holistic way. Biologists Harman and Sahtouris call for "a more holistic biology, characterized by recognition of the wholes being more than the sum of their parts, by 'emergent' qualities not reducible, even in principle, to the physical sciences."

*There is the synergy of nutrients and micronutrients*

Momma Nature is a spectacular provider of micronutrients that breast cancer survivors can add to their diets in combinations that have healing attributes, micronutrients that are strong by themselves, but become supercharged when combined with each other. We know that our biological systems never rely on just one micronutrient, but rather a system of micronutrients, for optimum performance.

I envision my task as providing as wide an array of combinations and permutations of plant nutrition as I possibly can, thereby increasing the chances that my body gets just what it needs to thrive. And so, each day, I mix it up, providing a full spectrum approach to nutrition meant to maximize the health of my organism.

*... and there is the synergy of how the nutrients are delivered*

It isn't just about taking this supplement or that. And dang-it-all I do want it be to be that easy, but it just isn't. Sorry, Dr. Oz fans: There is no miracle supplement. The true power of healing lies in the synergy of the actual food we use to nourish our bodies, by combining a wide variety of foods in a wide variety of ways that are now being shown to exponentially increase nutrient bioavailability.

I think that's the reductionism Harman and Sahtouris refer to: If we need more fiber, we eat more fiber-rich food and not just pop a mass-produced fiber tablet. For our vitamin D, we try to go outdoors and put our faces into the sun for a few minutes each day. (Unless, like me, you live in Michigan, in which case, we rely on supplements through the bleak gray winter.)

For our nutrients, we eat nutrient-rich whole foods, unless, of course, we are eating all the right things and are experiencing a deficiency that requires supplementation . . . the point being that we try to deliver our nutrients via food first and by supplementation last. (Work with your nutritionist to get this part right.)

I know, I know, different supplements have been thought to prevent or cure cancer, but listen up: Several trusted expert committees and scientific organizations have come to the conclusion that there is little to no scientific evidence that they do. Quite the contrary, there is now evidence that some supplements, such as beta-carotene, can actually increase cancer risk.

# ULTIMATE SURVIVORSHIP

*. . . and the synergy of keeping our bodies in motion,*
*of emotional well being, and of spiritual nourishment*

Once we have begun eating clean, healthy food, and avoiding the toxins that cause our bodies harm, we can't help but think about taking even more delight in our physical bodies, with gentle exercise that has been proven to be so beneficial in keeping recurrence at bay, and by loving ourselves truly and unconditionally, which, of course, builds on the holistic synergy of our new normal lives by easing our ability to keep our weight in a healthy range, which puts a big smile on our faces, which creates joy and love, which draws our loved ones near, old, new, and ancient alike, which blesses us with the support we need to help see us through to another year, which bolsters our strength in the face of adversity, which gives us the ability to climb tall mountains and to deny cancer a foothold, which provides us the fuel to pay it forward to others who are experiencing the pain we know so intimately, which helps to create an existence that is fundamentally deep and spiritual and absolutely, positively worth living.

*. . . and in conclusion*

My dear sisters, when I finally return to the stardust from whence I came, whether that moment is tomorrow or forty years from now, I want some-one telling the story of my life to start like this: "Once upon a time I knew a messy and imperfect and wild and joyful woman whose fondest desire was to grow old. Her name was Christine and she lived her life as best it could be imagined. She loved being alive and fully knew that each breath was an unearned gift from the universe. She was deeply present in her own life, and, when she was with me, she was deeply present in mine."

And I will ask you in closing: What is your fondest desire? It's time to start creating the future that only you can imagine. Peace to you and peace in your heart. I'm glad you are here.

*With all my love, Christine*

# AFTERWORD

I was blessed with a substantial contingent of friends and family who took the time to read my manuscript, and to a person, I was told that there were blanks left to be filled in. And honestly, I'm okay with that. This book is not intended to provide you with all of the information you will ever need on the topic of Your Breast Cancer, but rather, is to be used as a springboard of information that will lead you to ask specific questions from your breast care team.

If I had only one goal in mind for publishing this material, it would be that you empower yourself to ask questions of the people in whom you have entrusted your life. Ask questions until you are done asking them.

I am telling the absolute truth when I report that, at the time this book first neared completion, it contained almost 30,000 more words than it does today: *Ultimate Survivorship* was a lumbering behemoth crammed to the margins with details, details, and more details. (Actually, that was an entire section of the book, and that's exactly what it was called.)

It would have cost more to produce and distribute and would have required that I increase the price of the book, something I didn't want to do. More importantly, I realized that much of the information that got edited out could be put online, especially the information that tends to be more fluid and likely to change.

The whole time I was researching and writing, an idea began to take hold that I would like to have an online presence, a place where my readers could stay current on what's happening on any given day in the breast cancer community. It grew from that idea into a website. It is my fervent hope that it continues to grow into a fountain of information for breast cancer survivors.

To that end, please go to www.ultimatesurvivorship.com to connect with the highest quality and most up-to-date information available.

## What will you find at www.ultimatesurvivorship.com?

· a detailed list of what's in my pantry

· Discussions of my favorite things, including more recipes from some of my favorite plant-strong bloggers and other chefs, my top ten (ish) favorite cookbooks, and the best-of-the-best healthy food blogs to inspire you in the kitchen

· up-to-date contact information for the organizations discussed in this book

· a couple of reading lists

· up-to-the-minute news from the breast cancer community

· photos and stories of inspiration and hope

· references for the material presented here

· and always, always, where you find me, you will find LOVE


I look forward to seeing you there

and on Facebook!

# STARTER RECIPES

Exploring new options,
experimenting with new ideas,
eating interesting new foods.

*"If we don't change, we don't grow. If we don't grow, we are not really living.
Growth demands a temporary surrender of security."*

~ Gail Sheehy

# LIST OF RECIPES

There are three things I enjoy just about every day: A green smoothie, a super-gigantic salad, and antioxidant-rich green tea. For that reason, I think it's a swell idea to start the recipe section with my practically foolproof master recipes for each.

After that, I'm also providing basic instructions for some of my favorite everyday foods, hoping to give you a foothold in the whole foods, plant-based way of life. Finally, I'm including a penny-pinching recipe for a fruit and veggie wash that will help you avoid at least some of the contaminants found on your produce.

I also provide a list of amazing food blogs absolutely bursting with great food and the best introductory cookbooks for a whole foods, plant-based lifestyle at:

### *www.ultimatesurvivorship.com*

### *GREEN SMOOTHIE MASTER RECIPE - 1 serving*

1 c. leafy greens, torn up and packed down (kale, spinach, collards, chard)
1 c. fresh or frozen crucifer (broccoli, Brussels sprouts, etc.)
1 c. fresh or frozen fruit, mixed
½ banana (frozen) or avocado (not frozen)
1-3 T. freshly-ground flaxseed
1 T. protein powder (optional - not made with whey or soy)
2 c. water

Blend until frothy and delicious. This should make approximately one quart, perfect to take on the road in a wide-mouth mason jar. Start with more fruit than vegetables and slowly change the ratio as your taste buds change. If you aren't used to flaxseed yet, start with a small amount (a teaspoon) and build on that.

**Add-in extras** (all optional and all in small amounts): peanut butter, coconut flakes, dates, a splash of ginger juice or vanilla, cinnamon, spirulina powder, cocoa powder, xylitol or stevia if the protein powder is plain.

*Did you know that a canning jar with a regular size mouth*
*will fit perfectly onto most blender mechanisms?*
*Yeah, I know: Who knew?*
*Blend and go.*

**HUGH JASS SALAD MASTER RECIPE - 1 gigantic serving**

2 c. leafy greens (Romaine lettuce with any mixtures of greens, except iceberg)
1-3 c. chopped mixed color vegetables (cabbage, cauliflower, broccoli, tomatoes, onions, red pepper)
½ - 1 c. beans of any kind (kidney, butter, pinto, black: rinse well if canned)

**Add-in Extras** Chopped fruit and berries, dried fruit (my favorite are goji berries), and toasted sunflower or pumpkin seeds.

Gently toss in a giant salad bowl. Drizzle with the no-added fat salad dressing of your choice.

**Vinaigrette Dressing** Blend or whisk together ½ c. water, ¼ c. rice vinegar, ¼ c. red wine or apple cider vinegar, 2 cloves of garlic (minced small), 1 t. Italian seasoning, ¼ t. onion powder, 1 t. Bragg's Liquid Aminos, 2 t. xylitol or stevia, a bit of salt, a bit of pepper, a titch of turmeric.

**Creamy Ranch Dressing** Blend together ¼ package firm tofu, ¼ c. raw cashews (soaked in hot filtered water for at least an hour to add to their creaminess), 1 c. plain unsweetened nut milk, 2 T. lemon juice, 1 T. prepared mustard, ½ t. garlic powder, ½ t. onion powder, ½ t. dill weed, a bit of salt, a bit of pepper, and a dash of something hot, such as sriracha sauce or red pepper.

**Spicy Dressing** Blend together ½ c. rice vinegar, ½ c. salsa, 1 clove of garlic, a dash of lime juice, and ½ t. of cumin.

**Creamy Sunflower Seed Dressing** Blend together ½ c. plain unsweetened nut milk, ¼ c. tahini, ¼ c. lemon juice, a bit of salt, a bit of pepper.

**Salad in a jar variation** Put your dressing in the bottom of a wide-mouth quart-sized mason jar. Next, layer the more sturdy greens, such as kale. Then add your veggies and lettuce, followed by the beans. Haul this to work and throw in the fridge. When lunchtime rolls around, simply tip the whole thing into a bowl and enjoy. The dressing will even end up on top! (You could easily make five days' worth of lunches at one time. How much simpler could that be?)

**THE PERFECT CUP OF GREEN TEA - *1 serving***

½ t. loose-leaf green tea
7-8 ounces hot filtered water

In order to obtain maximum antioxidant power from your loose-leaf green tea, it is important for it to brew for ten minutes; it should then be consumed within an hour.

Place one-half teaspoon of loose-leaf green tea in a metal, cloth, paper, or ceramic infuser. (Please, no plastic! Hot Water+Plastic=Toxic)

Use fresh, filtered water that has been heated to about 180 degrees, which is below boiling. I wait until I can see that the water in the very bottom of the electric tea kettle (glass) is just starting to form bubbles but hasn't exploded into a dramatic frenzy. If you let it go too long and it starts to boil, simply let it sit for a minute to cool down before pouring.

Pour 7-8 ounces of water into the cup and let brew for ten minutes.

Add a splash of lemon or ginger juice to boost antioxidant power. I don't sweeten my tea, but if you wish to, use xylitol or stevia.

### OATS IN A JAR - 1 serving

I really don't know what it is about meals in a jar, but here it is, meal number three in a mason jar. (I think it's because I have a job with long hours and have to eat lots of meals at work, and a jar full of food is just so blasted easy.)

½ c. rolled oats
½ c. unsweetened nut milk
½ ripe banana, mashed up
½ c. blueberries
1 t. xylitol
1 t. chia seeds
½ t. cinnamon
1 T. chopped walnuts

Put everything except the nuts in a mason jar and give it a good shake. Put in the refrigerator overnight. In the morning, you can either eat it right out of the jar, cold, or you can heat it up in the microwave, which is my preference. Please remember to take the metal or plastic lid off the jar prior to microwaving! Add the chopped nuts right before you eat it.

*Variations* There are so many variations on this it's not even funny, including changing the fruit (chopped apples, cherries, peaches, oranges, as you wish) and adding different toppings, such as coconut, cacao nibs, cherries, granola, vanilla, or a drizzle of maple syrup. Or you could add three tablespoons of pureed pumpkin and some pumpkin pie spice with a few chopped pecans. Some people like to add non-dairy yogurt to their overnight oats (me, not-so-much).

## BUCKWHEAT BLUEBERRY PANCAKES - 4 to 6 servings

These are the pancakes my children ate just about every Sunday morning for most of their lives, over the years tweaked and fiddled with such that they are now fat-free and dairy-free. They're still mighty delicious.

### The dry ingredients

1 c. whole wheat flour or whole wheat pastry flour
¼ c. buckwheat flour
2 t. xylitol or coconut sugar
1 t. baking powder
½ t. baking soda

### The wet ingredients

1 c. unsweetened nut or flaxseed milk
½ t. organic distilled white vinegar
1 flaxseed egg (recipe on next page)
2 T. applesauce
½ c. blueberries

Mix the dry ingredients in a medium-sized bowl.

Place the milk in a second bowl and add the vinegar to it. Allow the milk to curdle for a few minutes, and then add the rest of the wet ingredients.

Add the wet to the dry ingredients, stirring just enough to combine them. Don't overstir. Let the batter rest for a few minutes to allow the baking soda to react with the curdled milk. Just before making the pancakes, gently fold in the blueberries.

Heat a well-seasoned cast-iron pan (or griddle) over medium heat. Pour 1/3 cup of batter onto the pan or griddle. Cook until you sneak a peek and see that the bottoms are nicely browned and bubbles appear on the top. Flip and cook until brown on the other side.

This is delicious with non-dairy yogurt and lightly drizzled with maple syrup. This recipe produces a fairly thick batter that holds up to additions very well. If you prefer a thinner batter, add a splash of water or nut milk and omit the blueberries in the batter. Serve with blueberries sprinkled on top instead of inside.

**Variations** Switch out the buckwheat flour with cornmeal, and the blueberries for corn. Switch out the buckwheat flour for brown rice flour, and the blueberries for fresh diced peaches, and garnished with toasted pecans.

### GROUND FLAXSEED (OR CHIA) EGG

This egg can be used 1:1 in any recipe calling for eggs as a binder. (But unfortunately you can't make scrambled eggs with them). If made properly, this is an excellent binder, just like eggs. Make sure you allow the full 15 minutes in the refrigerator that is called for, because if you don't, they will not perform nearly as beautifully as these.

1 T. freshly-ground flaxseed (or ground chia)
3 T. filtered water

Put the ground flaxseed in a small dish. Add the water to it. (Don't do it the other way around, you have to trust me on this.) Refrigerate for 15 minutes for maximum performance.

### SCRAMBLED EGGS

While I am on the topic of eggs, I thought I would share that there are several admirable substitutions that can be made for the scrambled variety. Vegans have a soft spot for this classic: Firm tofu with the water pressed out which is then scrambled with nooch (nutritional yeast) and spices. If you add a pinch of kala namak (natural black salt with a mild sulphur aroma and eggy flavor) it will taste even more like eggs.

### SCRAMBLED EGGS WITH GARBANZO BEAN FLOUR

There are many, many recipes out there for scrambled eggs made with garbanzo bean flour and spices. I think these are my favorite. Look one up and try it!

### EGG SALAD

This is a cinch to duplicate. I have really and truly served this to numerous people who would have sworn it was "real" egg salad. You'll need one package of firm tofu and all the things you usually put in your egg salad.

1 pkg. firm tofu, pressed dry
mayo, yellow mustard, chopped celery, onions, and pickle relish to taste
a pinch of kala namak (also known as black salt, very "eggy" in taste and aroma)
¼ teaspoon turmeric

Divide the tofu in two portions. Crumble one half like egg yolks and add turmeric to it to make it yellow. Dice the other half small and add the kala namak. Gently mix the two together and add the rest of the ingredients to taste.

*TEMPEH BREAKFAST STRIPS - makes 20-75 strips (I know, a very wide range, but it depends entirely on how thin you slice 'em . . . it's up to you)*

1 eight oz. pkg tempeh, sliced and steamed for 15 minutes
½ c. filtered water (for the marinade)
¼ c. low-sodium tamari (or Bragg's Liquid Aminos)
2 T. apple cider vinegar
1 T. coconut sugar or maple syrup
½ t. ground cumin
½ t. chili powder
½ t. turmeric
¼ t. smoked paprika
1 t. liquid smoke (optional)
a dash of cayenne powder (if you're feeling spicy)

Cut the tempeh as thin as you can with as sharp a knife as you own, across the short side of the block, making shorter strips. Steam the strips for 15 minutes.

While the tempeh is steaming, make the marinade by placing the water, tamari, apple cider vinegar, sweetener of choice, cumin, chili powder, and turmeric in a saucepan and bringing it to a boil. Turn off the heat and add liquid smoke, if using. Allow everything to cool.

Place the tempeh in a large, flat dish or plastic container. (If you are a using plastic container, take special care to cool your ingredients to room temperature, as Hot+Plastic=Toxic.) Pour the marinade over the tempeh slices, cover, and allow to marinate in the fridge for a minimum of two hours, but up to overnight.

When marinating is complete and you are ready to eat, preheat the oven to 325 degrees. Line a half-sheet baking pan first with aluminum foil and then parchment paper. (This will save scrubbing time later on.) Carefully place the tempeh slices in the pan and throw the marinade away. If you've done a great job cutting the slices thin, you may need to make two batches.

Sprinkle on the cayenne, if you are feeling spicy. Bake for 20 minutes, or until just starting to get brown. Flip them over with metal tongs, and bake for an additional 10 to 20 minutes, until crispy and fully browned.

These tend to get a little soft when stored. When eating them the second time, toast for 20 seconds in the microwave, or in a dry pan on the stove. The crunch will come back.

*Variations* You may also place the baking pans in the broiler on a low temperature, just be aware that they go from "almost-done" to "oops, too far" in a heartbeat. You can also dry-fry in a non-stick pan, as long as it is the newer, safer type of non-stick.

Eat right away with your blueberry buckwheat pancakes and save the leftovers for sandwiches and smoky, tasty crumbles for pizza.

### IMPORTANT NOTE ON COOKING WITH TEMPEH

Tempeh is one of the most versatile, high-protein ingredients in the refrigerator, and yet, one of the least-known in American kitchens. I'll never forget the first time I bought it (many moons ago) and immediately proceeded to cut off a chunk and pop it into my mouth, cold. It was not good (bitter and odd-tasting) and I was scared away from tempeh for many years after that.

I just didn't know what to do with it! While visiting a friend a few years later, I saw that she was steaming her tempeh, and when I asked why, she said it was to release bitterness and soften up the tempeh to accept her marinade. Eureka! I've never had bitter tempeh since that day.

Therefore, every recipe that calls for tempeh starts with steaming it for 15 minutes, either in a little metal veggie steamer on the stove or in a rice steamer. If I am making sandwich patties, I will first cut it into four portions (once the long way, like cutting a hamburger bun, and then in half).

If I am making sloppy joes or a burger substitute, I'll crumble it. If I am making bacon, I slice it like a little loaf of bread (long way or short way, doesn't matter). This makes sure there is maximum steamage, which provides for maximum deliciousness.

**THE GENTLE CHEF'S BASIC SEITAN AND BEAF SEITAN** - Makes about 1¼ lb.
*From the Gentle Chef Cookbook by Skye Michael Conroy. Used with permission.*

Basic and beaf seitan are essentially the same, except beaf seitan contains an additional ingredient to enhance color and is simmered in a "beef"-flavored broth, rather than a basic vegetable broth. "Beaf" is a word derived from the consonants of the word "beef" and the vowels of the word "wheat."

Seitan can be shaped in many ways prior to simmering, depending upon its intended application; the shaping techniques are explained in the recipe.

For the best texture, simmered beaf seitan should be refrigerated for a minimum of eight hours before final preparation; so plan accordingly.

*Sift together the following dry ingredients in a large mixing bowl:*
1 c. vital wheat gluten
2 T. garbanzo bean (chickpea) flour
1 t. onion powder
1 t. garlic powder
¼ t. ground white pepper

*For the liquid ingredients, mix the following in a separate bowl or measuring cup:*
3/4 c. water
2 T. nutritional yeast
1 T. tamari, soy sauce, or Bragg's Liquid Aminos
1 T. vegetable oil
1 t. Gravy Master or other browning liquid (for beaf seitan)

*For the simmering broth you will need:*
6 c. vegetable broth (for basic seitan)
*or*
6 c. beaf broth (for beaf seitan)

**Technique** In a large sauce pan, set your broth over high heat while you pre-pare your seitan dough. You will want to bring it to a rapid boil. Add the liquid ingredients (but not the simmering broth!) to the dry ingredients in a large bowl and mix well.

Turn out onto a work surface and knead vigorously with the heel of your hand for several minutes to develop the gluten. The dough will become very elastic. Now, you will need to shape the dough prior to simmering, and there are dif-ferent ways to do this, depending upon your desired application.

**If you need thin slices,** form the dough into a rounded loaf shape and cut in half with a sharp knife. Simmer and refrigerate as directed, then slice thin.

*If you intend to later thread your seitan onto skewers for grilling*, divide the dough into six to nine equal pieces. Squeeze and shape the pieces into slender 3 or 4-inch long "tenders" and slightly flatten them with the palm of your hand. Simmer and refrigerate as directed, then skewer.

*For "steak" cutlets*, which can later be cut into strips if desired, divide the dough into four to six pieces. Stretch and flatten each piece with the heel of your hand. Let rest for a few minutes and then flatten again to form very thin cutlets. Simmer and refrigerate as directed, then use in your intended recipe.

*Back to the main recipe for all applications* Next, add the shaped dough to the boiling broth. The addition of the dough may temporarily halt the boiling action. Once the broth begins to bubble again, immediately adjust the heat to a gentle, lazy simmer and set the timer for 45 minutes. Be sure to leave the pot uncovered. If you've divided the dough into strips or cutlets, simmer for 30 minutes.

The first 10 minutes of simmering is the most crucial, as this is when the texture is set. Watch the pot and continue to adjust the heat by increments, up or down as necessary, to maintain a gentle simmer. If you catch the broth rapidly simmering, reduce the heat slightly. Turn occasionally once the seitan pieces float to the top of the pot.

When finished cooking, remove the pot from the heat and let the seitan cool in the broth until it reaches room temperature. It will be very soft at this point. Refrigerate the seitan with about ¼ cup of the simmering broth in a leak-proof plastic bag or airtight container for a minimum of eight hours, or for up to 10 days, before final preparation. This will form the seitan and optimize its texture. You can also freeze it for up to three months.

Reserve the remaining broth for other uses, but be sure to add back a little water if necessary, as the broth may have become very salty from evaporation during simmering.

*Final preparation and uses for Basic and Beef Seitan* Larger pieces are at their best when sliced very thin and pan-seared. They can also be finely diced. The slices and dices hold up very well in hearty soups, stews, and pot pies. Try thin-slicing simmered seitan and serve with BBQ sauce on a bun; or glaze with teriyaki sauce and serve over rice. Pan-sear seitan cutlets, then slice into thin strips for "steak" sandwiches. Cutlets may also be breaded or used in shish-kabob or satay. Ground beef seitan is an excellent alternative for any dish calling for pre-cooked and crumbled ground beef. Simply cut the chunks and grind in a food processor.

### CRAZY AND DELICIOUS CARROT DOGS - 4 servings

Summertime and the living is easy. Grilled corn and zucchini, fresh strawberries, and crazy, delicious hot dogs . . . made out of carrots? I can hear you all the way over here: Are you kidding me, Christine? I am telling you right here, that if I hadn't cooked them myself, there is just no way in the world I would have guessed it. (I fooled Mr. Anderson as well.) This version is an adaptation of a recipe found on the Fatfree Vegan blog, who originally found it on the Healthy Slow Cooking blog, and which I (of course) tweaked to suit my tastes.

4 big organic carrots, cut into bun lengths and shaped into dogs
¼ c. filtered water
3 T. Bragg's Liquid Aminos
3 T. seasoned rice vinegar
1 t. Liquid Smoke
¼ t. granulated garlic powder
¼ t. ground ginger
1/8 t. onion powder
freshly-ground pepper to taste (please, no salt, it's in the Bragg's)

Fill a pot with water and heat to boiling. Turn down to medium and add the carrots. Cook until you can just pierce one with a fork but it still has a little snap to it. Dump them in cold (ice) water to halt the cooking process.

While the carrots are cooking, prepare the marinade by whisking everything but the carrots together in a container that will allow the carrots to lay flat and won't leak when you roll them around while marinating.

Place the cooled carrots in the container, give a little shake, and let them marinade for a minimum of 3 hours, but up to a few days. Turn over or shake from time to time.

To serve, cook in a nonstick or cast iron skillet, or on a medium-hot grill, until heated through. It'll take about 10-15 minutes. Serve just like any other hot dog, with all the fixins you enjoy. Not just crazy, not just delicious . . . but crazy delicious!

### AMAZON BURGERS - 6 to 9 servings

We can't have hot dogs without burgers, and the Amazon is just what is called for! This recipe was given to me by a friend, who got it from a friend who remembered the recipe from working at "this really cool restaurant that closed years ago in Ann Arbor." It's a bit of a pain to make, with all of the chopping, but I'm telling you, it's worth it times a bazillion. (Or use a food processor.)

3/4 c. dry plain lentils (the mushy kind, not the French kind)
1½ c. water
2 T. filtered water
1 c. finely chopped onion
4-5 large cloves garlic, finely minced
1 red bell pepper, finely chopped
1 medium carrot, peeled and finely chopped
2 celery stalks, finely chopped
8-10 large baby bella mushrooms, finely chopped
½ c. minced walnuts
2 flaxseed eggs
¼ c. overcooked pasta, blended
½ c. bread crumbs
1 t. dry mustard powder
1 t. chili powder
2 t. Bragg's Liquid Aminos
½ t. freshly-ground black pepper (please, no salt, it's in the Bragg's)
1 t. sriracha (hot sauce)

Sort through the lentils for stones. Place lentils and water in a small saucepan and bring to a boil. Lower heat and simmer, covered, for about 30 minutes, or until the lentils are soft and the liquid is gone. Transfer to a mixing bowl. Drain if needed.

Chop your veggies (or process with a food processor) while the lentils are cooking. Heat the water in a large skillet. Add onions and sauté on medium heat for about 5 minutes. Add garlic in the last minute. Add the remaining veggies and cook for about 10 minutes so the mushrooms release their juices and veggies are tender. Add the seasonings, stir, and taste. If everything is tender, transfer to the lentil bowl. If not, cook some more.

Mix in the blended overcooked pasta, the flax eggs, and the bread crumbs. Chill for about an hour to firm up. Mix the whole thing with your hands, and form into patties. I usually use about 1/3 of a cup per burger. Sauté in a nonstick or cast iron skillet for 5-8 minutes per side.

### *OH-MY-GOSH BEANY BROTHY DELICIOUSNESS (OMG BBD)*
From The Recipe Renovator blog by Stephanie Weaver. Used with permission.

2 c. (1 lb or 450 g) dried beans
3 carrots, any size
4 stalks celery
1 white, yellow, or brown onion
2 cloves garlic
2 sweet potatoes, optional
fennel tops (3-5 fronds)
thyme sprigs (a handful or a package)
2 bay leaves
up to 2 T. kosher salt (omit or reduce for low-sodium version)
1 T. organic extra-virgin olive oil (use the good stuff, please)
8 c. filtered or spring water

Pour out the dry beans into a shallow bowl, a bit at a time, and pick through them. Remove any pebbles, sticks, or discolored beans. Some people remove broken beans. I'm not that picky. But yes, I've found pebbles before so don't skip this step.

Put the sorted beans in a large pot and rinse and swirl with enough water to cover them. I use tap water for this step. Drain completely.

Cover the beans with enough *filtered* water to allow them to double in size. Leave on the counter overnight.

In the morning, rinse and drain the beans. Return them to the cooking pot.

Prep the vegetables and add them to the pot as you go:

· Scrub the carrots and celery, cut off the tops and bottoms, and cut into three large chunks.

· Cut off the stem end of the onion, then cut it in half lengthwise through the root end. Peel off the papery skin. If you want onions in with your beans at the end, slice the onion lengthwise. If you want the beans to go off and have another beany life in a different recipe, quarter the onion.

· Smash the garlic cloves with the flat blade of your chef's knife. Kapow! Remove the papery skin.

· Scrub the potatoes, peel if desired, and cut into large chunks or small dice. (If you want potato dice in your beans at the end, dice the potatoes. If you want to be able to fish the pieces out, cut into quarters.)

· Tie the washed fennel fronds and thyme sprigs into a bundle with some clean kitchen twine.

· Add the bay leaves, salt, olive oil, and filtered water.

Bring just to a boil with the lid on the pot, then turn down to a simmer (just barely bubbling). Check the beans after 30 minutes. You want them to be nicely tender but not falling apart. If you are going to make baked beans, you want them to still be pretty firm. Depending on the size of the beans, they cook in 30-120 minutes.

Once the beans are done, remove the herb bundle and bay leaves and compost them. Fish out the large chunks of veggies with a slotted spoon. You can mash those up for a puree, or blend them with some of the Brothy Deliciousness (BD) and make a lovely veggie soup the next day. Drain the extra BD into a container. Use it to make gravy or use it instead of water to cook rice, quinoa, or millet, for more OMG deliciousness.

Serve the drained beans as is, or use them in any recipe calling for cooked beans.

## HOW TO COOK ANY GRAIN
*Courtesy of Oldways Preservation Trust and the Whole Grains Council,*
*www.wholegrainscouncil.org. Used with permission.*

You can add whole grains to your meals without cooking, simply by choosing breads, breakfast cereals, and other prepared whole grain foods. If you'd like to enjoy delicious whole grains at home as a side dish, however, here are some guidelines for cooking them from scratch.

*Plain grain, general directions* Cooking most grains is very similar to cooking rice. You put the dry grain in a pan with water or broth; bring it to a boil, then simmer until the liquid is absorbed. Pasta is generally cooked in a larger amount of water; the excess is drained away after cooking. Don't be intimidated!

*Grain pilaf, general directions* Caramelize small bits of onion, mushroom, and garlic in a little bit of broth in a sauce pan. Add grain and cook briefly, coating the grains in the caramelized vegetables; then add broth in the amount specified in the chart that follows, and cook until liquid is absorbed.

*Important: time varies* Grains can vary in cooking time depending on the age of the grain, the variety, and the pan you are using to cook. When you decide they are tender and tasty, they're done! If the grain is not as tender as you like when "time is up," simply add more water and continue cooking. Or, if everything seems fine before the liquid is absorbed, simply drain the excess.

*Shortcut* If you want to cook grains more quickly, simply let them sit in the allotted amount of water for a few hours before cooking. Just before dinner, add extra water, if necessary; then cook. You'll find that cooking time is much shorter with a little pre-soaking. *Another shortcut* is to cook whole grains in big batches. Grains keep three to four days in the fridge and take just minutes to warm up with a little added water or broth. You can also use the leftovers for cold salads (just toss with chopped veggies, dressing, and anything else that suits your fancy), or toss a few handfuls in some soup. Cook once and then take it easy.

*Sticky bottoms* If whole grains are sticking to the bottom of the pan, turn off the heat, add a very small amount of liquid, stick a lid on the pan, and let it sit a few minutes. The grain will loosen, easing serving and cleanup.

*Nuttier, fuller flavor* Whole grains are generally chewier than refined grains and have a nuttier, fuller flavor. You may find this unfamiliar at first, but after a month or two, refined grains may start to taste very plain and uninteresting by contrast. Stick with it until your palate adjusts, and reap the health benefits.

## *WHOLE GRAIN COOKING CHART*

| To 1 cup of this grain: | Add this much water or broth: | Bring to a boil, then simmer for: | Amount after cooking: |
|---|---|---|---|
| Amaranth | 2 cups | 20-25 minutes | 3½ cups |
| Barley, hulled | 3 cups | 45-60 minutes | 3½ cups |
| Buckwheat | 2 cups | 20 minutes | 4 cups |
| Bulgur | 2 cups | 10-12 minutes | 3 cups |
| Cornmeal (polenta) | 4 cups | 25-30 minutes | 2½ cups |
| Couscous, whole wheat | 2 cups | 10 minutes (heat off) | 3 cups |
| Kamut® grain | 4 cups | Soak overnight, then cook 45-60 minutes | 3 cups |
| Millet, hulled | 2½ cups | 25-35 minutes | 4 cups |
| Oats, steel cut | 4 cups | 20 minutes | 4 cups |
| Pasta, whole wheat | 6 cups | 8-12 minutes (varies by size) | Varies |
| Quinoa | 2 cups | 12-15 minutes | 3+ cups |
| Rice, brown | 2½ cups | 25-45 minutes (varies by variety) | 3-4 cups |
| Rye berries | 4 cups | Soak overnight, then cook 45-60 minutes | 3 cups |
| Sorghum | 4 cups | 25-40 minutes | 3 cups |
| Spelt berries | 4 cups | Soak overnight, then cook 45-60 minutes | 3 cups |
| Wheat berries | 4 cups | Soak overnight, then cook 45-60 minutes | 3 cups |
| Wild rice | 3 cups | 45-55 minutes | 3½ cups |

*Courtesy of Oldways Preservation Trust and the Whole Grains Council, www.wholegrainscouncil.org. Used with permission.*

### GRILLED PORTOBELLO STEAKS

Portobello mushrooms have a wonderfully deep and rich taste; the firm, chewy texture makes them a perfect centerpiece for a meal that used to feature ingredients no longer on our shopping lists. It's no wonder they are the steak of the veggie world!

4 large Portobello mushroom caps
3 T. finely minced onion
4 T. finely minced garlic
4 T. apple cider vinegar
1 T. low-sodium tamari (or Bragg's Liquid Aminos)
1 t. Monterey seasoning

Put all of the marinade ingredients in a container that won't leak when you shake it. Twist and pop the stems off the mushroom caps, and place the caps in the marinade. Cover, shake, and marinate for up to an hour.

Grill for 5 minutes on each side. Serve as you would a burger, on a toasted bun with vegan Swiss cheese, caramelized onions, and a slice of tomato.

### NON-FAT CARAMELIZED ONIONS

1 large onion (any kind, and cut as you wish)
1 t. salt
filtered water, as needed

Place the onion in a large pan along with the salt and any other seasonings you'd like to add. Note: Do not omit the salt, as this is crucial for drawing the water out of the onions and is an important part of the caramelization process without added fat!

Cover the pan and turn the heat to low to draw most of the water out of the onions, which will take up to 15 minutes. Pay attention to the cooking process and don't allow it to go too quickly.

Uncover the pan and keep on cooking until the water has reduced almost completely and the onions start to darken to a deep golden hue: Caramelization magic has occurred! Watching carefully, turn the heat up to medium-high and add water, about ½ cup, stirring to deglaze the tasty brown bits that are now forming. Do not let it burn. (Not tasty.)

Keep adding ½ cup of water to almost-dry onions as needed, stopping when the onions reach the level of sweetness and softness that you prefer.

## *NONFAT TOFU & VEGGIE STEAM-FRY MASTER RECIPE*

Use a well-seasoned wok or a giant cast iron skillet and heat it up prior to starting the stir fry. All you have to do is substitute water for oil at the moment it's go-time.

½ large onion, sliced into thin strips
6 cups of mixed vegetables, cut into similar-size chunks
1 block of firm or extra firm tofu, pressed
a squirt of low-sodium tamari or Bragg's Liquid Aminos

**Add-ons** Toasted peanuts, pepitas, sunflower seeds, or walnuts. Add extra water or broth or light coconut milk and a teaspoon of red curry paste. Thicken with a tablespoon of cornstarch in a half cup of cold liquid. Add a tablespoon of chopped ginger (see note below) or a couple of shakes of ginger juice. Add a teaspoon of turmeric! (My favorite. I love to turn my food yellow.)

**Equipment**
Tofu press or homemade contraption
Wok or large cast iron skillet with a fitted lid

Press your block of tofu. You can use an actual piece of kitchen apparatus called a tofu press, or, if you are like me and don't own one of those, you can improvise by wrapping the block of tofu in two clean flour-sack towels and precariously balancing a couple of heavy objects (2-3 pounds) on a plate set directly on top of it. If you don't have flour-sack towels, check them out! They are like paper towels, but made of cloth. This balancing act can also account for the entertainment portion of the evening.

**Hint** Stack it in a corner, and not near an edge. Press for a minimum of one hour (or up to four hours, to get it good and dry) using your homemade contraption. If you own a tofu press, follow the instructions that came with it.

Heat up the broiler, on high. Cover a half-sheet or cookie pan with aluminum foil. You may wish to use a very light spray of extra-virgin olive oil at this point. (I don't usually as aluminum foil is pretty nonstick.)

Cut the pressed tofu into chunks and place on the prepared pan. Broil until nice and crispy on the top side. Turn over with kitchen tongs (or just stir them up) and continue broiling until they're done. Set aside.

Heat up the wok or cast iron skillet, toss the water or broth in, and cook the onions until translucent, stirring frequently and adding more liquid as needed. Add the ginger and continue stirring for 1 minute. Toss in the rest of the vegetables, adding more liquid as necessary, a tablespoon at a time, steam-frying for another minute. Add the tofu chunks. Squirt tamari or Bragg's onto every-thing and put the lid on. Turn the heat off and let it steam for another minute.

Serve on top of a cup of brown rice or your favorite noodles. Garnish each serving with a teaspoon of toasted nuts.

**Ginger hint** I don't think I'm alone in saying that I have a hard time keeping fresh ginger fresh. It always goes bad before I finish a knuckle of it! And peeling ginger has never been good times for me. I now have two tricks for that, and rarely buy fresh anymore. One is ginger juice from the Ginger People, and the other is candied ginger. I know, it's covered in sugar. But. Spend a few seconds rubbing that ginger under warm running water, and you get the softest, not-sweet except in a really terrific way, piece of ginger, that you could imagine.

### ENDURANCE CRACKERS - *22 large crackers*
*From OhSheGlows.com by Angela Liddon. Used with permission.*

These crackers are extremely light and crispy while providing long-lasting energy. They are also dairy-free, gluten-free, soy-free, nut-free, sugar-free and oil-free to boot! Feel free to change up the seasonings and spices as you wish. Herbamare is a delicious organic salt blend; kelp granules add a "taste of the sea" to your recipes. Both can be found in health food stores.

½ c. chia seeds
½ c. sunflower seeds
½ c. pepitas (pumpkin seeds)
½ c. sesame seeds
1 c. water
1 large garlic clove, finely grated
1 t. grated sweet onion
¼ t. kosher salt, or to taste
Herbamare and kelp granules, to taste (optional)

Preheat the oven to 325 degrees and line a large baking sheet with parchment paper.

In a large bowl, mix the seeds together. In a small bowl, mix the water, grated garlic, and grated onion. Whisk well. Pour the water mixture onto the seeds and stir until thick and combined. Season with salt and optional Herbamare and kelp granules to taste. Add spices or fresh herbs if you wish.

Spread the mixture onto the prepared baking sheet with the back of a spoon until it's less than ¼ inch thick. Not to worry if a couple parts become too thin, you can just patch them up.

Bake for 30 minutes. Remove from oven, slice into crackers. Carefully flip onto other side with a spatula. Bake for another 30 minutes, watching closely after about 25 minutes. The bottoms will be lightly golden in color. Allow to cool completely on the pan. Store in an airtight container.

Delicious as-is or with no-added-fat hummus.

**VANILLA CHIA PUDDING - 8 servings**
*Adapted from a recipe found at MarthaStewart.com.*

½ c. chia seeds
4 t. vanilla extract
1 c. raw cashews, soaked in hot filtered water for 1-3 hours
6-8 Medjool dates (to taste), pits removed
4 c. filtered water
2 T. coconut sugar
pinch of sea salt
¼ t. ground garam masala (or cinnamon)
2 c. mixed berries (raspberries, blueberries, blackberries)
maple syrup, for drizzling

Drain cashews and rinse well. Place them in a blender along with the filtered water, dates, garam masala, and vanilla extract. Blend on high for two minutes and pour into a bowl with the chia seeds. Whisk well. Let the pudding stand for 15 minutes, making sure to whisk every few minutes to prevent the chia seeds from clumping together.

Refrigerate until cold. Serve with fruit sprinkled on top and drizzled with maple syrup and a dollop of Coconut Milk Creamy Whipped. Add cocoa nibs, or pureed berries, or chunks of fruit and other spices, to change up this nutritious and filling snack or dessert.

## COCONUT MILK CREAMY WHIPPED TOPPING

I usually keep a can of coconut milk in the fridge so I am always prepared to make this delicious, creamy whipped topping, which is excellent on fresh berries, cupcakes, or chia pudding.

1 can full fat coconut milk (this will not work with light versions)
1 T. xylitol or stevia
1 t. vanilla extract
1 T. cornstarch

Chill the coconut milk in the refrigerator overnight.

About an hour before actual preparation, place metal bowl and beaters in the freezer to chill.

If the xylitol is made of large crystals (as it often is), grind it in a spice grinder to a fine powder. Open the bottom of the coconut milk can; carefully, slowly, pour the coconut milk into another container (reserve for use in a smoothie or add to soup or to steam-fried veggies with some red curry paste). What's left in the can will be full-fat coconut cream.

Whip it. Whip it good. (Along with the vanilla and the cornstarch, in the cold container and with the cold beaters.)

This is not a low-fat dessert item and is a true indulgence, from time to time.

### *CASHEW BUTTER*

Cashew butter is the main ingredient in any number of healthy whole-food plant-based recipes, including sour cream, cashew milk, cheezy sauces, a wonderful heavy cream substitute, and much, much more. You can purchase it at your health food store or online, but it tends to be a bit expensive.

It's easy enough to make on your own, and only requires one ingredient: Raw unsalted cashews. There are many recipes for cashew butter that make use of added oil and liquid sweeteners, but resist the urge to add anything but the nuts, and possibly a tiny amount of salt, to taste.

Place two to four cups of cashews in your high-powered blender (or in a food processor). Process slowly, taking breaks to let your machine cool down if it gets hot, as this is not a speedy process. It will go from nut chunks, to small pieces, to flour, to a big ball of dry nuts. Don't panic when it gets to this place. Stay with it; hang tight! Continue processing and taking breaks until finally, the butter is quite warm and begins to release its own oils, is sweet, creamy, and delicious. Store in glass jars.

### *CASHEW SOUR CREAM SAUCE*
*From The Ultimate Uncheese Cookbook by Jo Stepaniak. Used with permission.*

Try this delectable, creamy sauce on potatoes, noodles, vegetables, or grains. It's the perfect sour cream replacement for breast cancer survivors! Use cold water for a cold sauce, or hot water for an instant, no-cook warm sauce.

½ c. cashew butter
2 T. fresh lemon juice
salt
1 c. hot or cold water, more or less as needed

Combine all ingredients in a blender or food processor, using just enough water to make a thick, smooth sauce. Alternatively, combine all ingredients, except water, in a small bowl. Gradually stir in enough water to make a thick but pourable sauce.

### EASY-PEASY SPREADABLE CHEEZY

This is great on sandwiches or crackers. And when I say it's easy to make, I'm not just whistlin' Dixie, sister. I make this with garbanzo bean flour, that I toast in a pan on the stove first, which imparts great flavor to the Cheezy. You can substitute just about any flour you have on hand.

**Blend:**
½ c. fire-roasted red peppers
½ c. garbanzo bean flour
½ c. nooch (nutritional yeast)
1 c. filtered water
3 T. tahini
2 T. lemon juice
1 t. salt

Pour into a lightly coated loaf pan. Bake at 350 degrees for about 30 minutes, until it's firm in the center.

### *CHUNKY ROQUEFORT DIP AND DRESSING*

*From The Ultimate Uncheese Cookbook by Jo Stepaniak. Used with permission.*

¼ pound (4 ounces) firm regular tofu, drained
1½ c. (about 12 ounces) crumbled firm silken tofu
½ c. plain nondairy milk
1 T. sesame tahini
4 t. umeboshi plum paste
1 t. nutritional yeast flakes
½ to 1 t. crushed garlic
a pinch of white pepper
1 T. minced fresh parsley, or 1½ t. dried parsley

Break the regular tofu into large chunks. Place in a saucepan and cover with water. Bring to a boil, reduce heat, and simmer 5 minutes. Drain well. Chill uncovered in the refrigerator until cool enough to handle. Crumble and set aside. Place remaining ingredients, except parsley, in a food processor and process until very smooth and creamy. Mixture will be very thick. Briefly pulse-in the parsley and reserved tofu, keeping the tofu in small to mid-sized chunks. Chill several hours or overnight before serving to allow flavors to blend. This should keep for five to seven days in the refrigerator.